cl

A Colour Atlas of Contact Lenses
(& Prosthetics)

A Colour Atlas of
Contact Lenses
(& Prosthetics)

Professor Montague Ruben

FRCS

Consultant Ophthalmologist and Director
Dept. Contact Lens and Prosthetics
Moorfields Eye Hospital
London
also
Visiting Professor
Dept. Optometry
The City University
London

Wolfe Medical Publications Ltd

Copyright © M. Ruben, 1982
Published by Wolfe Medical Publications Ltd, 1982
Printed by Royal Smeets Offset b.v., Weert, Netherlands
ISBN 0 7234 0774 6

This book is one of the titles in the series of
Wolfe Medical Atlases, a series which brings
together probably the world's largest systematic
published collection of diagnostic colour
photographs.
For a full list of Atlases in the series, plus
forthcoming titles and details of our surgical,
dental and veterinary Atlases, please write to
Wolfe Medical Publications Ltd, Wolfe House,
3 Conway Street, London W1P 6HE.

General Editor, Wolfe Medical Atlases:
G. Barry Carruthers, MD(Lond)

Contents

3 Clinical cases (including therapeutic)

References

Ruben M (1975) *'Textbook of Contact Lens Practice'* Bailliere Tindall, London
Ruben M (ed) (1978) *'Soft Lenses'* Bailliere Tindall, London, & J Wiley Inc., New York

Further reading:

Bier N & Lowther J (1977) *'Contact Lens Corrections'* Butterworths, London
Stone J & Phillips A (1980) *'Contact Lenses'* vols I & II Butterworths, London
Mandell R (1979) *'Contact Lens Practice'* Springfield, Illinois, Thomas

Abbreviations

A.E.L., (ζ), ($\int$) = Axial Edge Lift
Ax = Axial Power of eye
BCOD = Back Central Optic Diameter
BCOR = Back Central Optic Radius
BVD = Back Vertex Distance
CAB = Cellulose acetyl butyrate
E = Eccentricity
F = Focal Power f = focal length
K = Keratometry
O/S = Overall Size
OC = Over Correction (spectacle correction over contact lens)
PHEMA = Polyhydroxyethylmethacrylate
PMMA = Polymethylmethacrylate
$\underline{N}$ Saline = Physiological Saline (0.9%)
SPK = Superficial Punctate Keratitis
TD = Total lens diameter (also O/S)
$T°$ = Temperature
Tc = Centre lens thickness
Te = Edge lens thickness
T or t = Thickness
$\triangle$ = Prism dioptre

'It is the mark of the educated man to look for precision in each class of things so far as the nature of the subject admits.'

Aristotle
(Nichomachean Ethics)

Preface

Contact lens practice has changed radically in the last quarter of a century. However, unlike many advances in therapy where new procedures replace the old, contact lenses from each phase of development still remain in current practice. Each technological development has not produced, as yet, a contact lens which resolves all optical and physiological problems. Thus, although materials in all degrees of hardness and of the highest gas permeation may be available eventually, they may not be necessarily the material of choice to help a certain individual see well and provide a lifetime of use without adverse tissue reactions. Conversely, many conditions of the eye associated with disease may not be best suited to lenses specifically designed for the low myopic. The latter provide the bulk of cosmetic visual contact lens practice and the energy spent in the research and development of lenses for this type of patient far exceeds that of their use in other conditions.

This atlas therefore is a history of both the last few decades and also of current practice. It is impossible on the manufacturing side to but hint at the procedures. This book is intended for the clinical student practitioner as an aid to the conventional textbook. The latter very often has a minimal content of coloured pictures. It is impossible to cover the theory in an atlas and this must be learnt from comprehensive texts or from teachers.

This atlas may be useful for those practitioners who wish to specialise in contact lens practice or for ophthalmologists, optometrists and opticians who wish to understand better the extent of the practice. The many diverse uses of the contact lens and some examples of prosthetics are illustrated.

The photographs have been collected over several years and most patients were treated by myself at Moorfields Eye Hospital, many of the diagrams formed the bases of lectures or papers and were prepared by the Medical Illustration Department at the Institute of Ophthalmology, London (artist, Mr. Tarrant). New diagrams have been prepared by the publisher's artist. Some photographs and illustrations are printed by kind permission of the contributors, and they are gratefully acknowledged in the text.

I should like to thank Miss Margaret Ryder who helped take many of the earlier photographs and Sarah Harding who typed the legends.

I am indebted to past and present ophthalmological, optical, and technical members of the Moorfields Contact Lens Department for their help with both National Health and private patients; their interest is reflected in the following pages.

1. The material and lens

Physicochemical properties

1   Some contact lens materials.

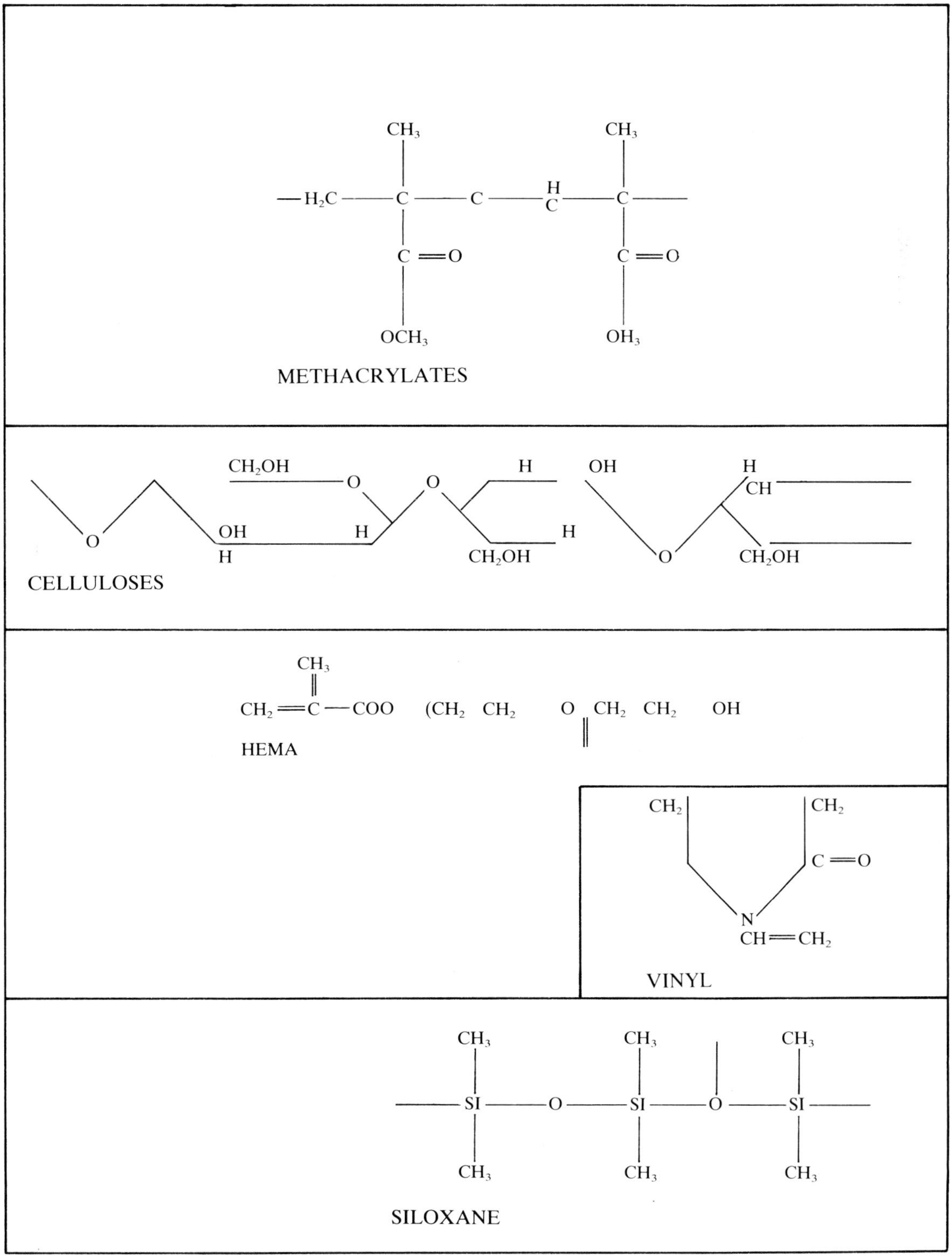

METHACRYLATES

CELLULOSES

HEMA

VINYL

SILOXANE

2   Lens fitting and wearing behaviour can be assessed from the following:

specific gravity
micro-penetration (hardness)
elasticity
plasticity
tensile strength
water absorption
surface wettability
stress and strain
gas permeability
thermal conductivity
coefficients of size relative to T^o (linear expansion)
coefficients of size relative to water (linear expansion)
refractive index
optical quality
light transmission %
gas permeability of lens relative to thickness
material purity
polymer stability etc.

3   Polymethylmethacrylate (PMMA) specifications. Example of USA material specifications for PMMA used in contact lens manufacture.

Specific gravity	1.18–1.19
Refractive index	1.49–1.50
Tensile strength	7000–9000
Hardness	M80–M100
Heat distribution T°	160–195°C
Polymerisation shrinkage volume	6%
Water absorption in 3mm specimen	0.20–0.50% in 24 hours

4 Design of lens size and thickness relative to physical properties.

Material	Relative hardness	Water content %	Relative gas (O_2) permeability	Surface wettability angle	Optimal lens size	Average thickness (mm)
PMMA	1.00	1	0	70–50°	7–12	0.12
CAB*	0.80	3	3–6	70–50°	9–12	0.12
Siloxane–acrylo-butyrates*	0.80–0.60	1–3	6–9	30–20°	9–13	0.12
Silicone rubber	0.050	0	100	90–50°	11–13	0.20
PHEMA and copolymers*	0.030	26–38	9–25	60°	12–15	0.10
Vinyl hemas*	0.020	45–70	25–60	40°	12–15	0.12
Amydo amines*	0.015	75	60	40°	13–15	0.20
Vinyls*	0.010	80	60+	40°	13–15	0.20

*Gas permeability is T° and thickness dependent. Wetting angles – regression and advanced angles for hard materials.
N.B. Actual centre and edge thickness is power dependent.

5   The rigid lens (or hard lens) – definition.

A lens that with normal lid pressure, body temperature and water content at equilibrium with the wearing environment *does not mould* to the eye surface.

6   The soft lens – definition.

A lens that with normal lid pressure, body temperature and water content at equilibrium with the wearing environment does mould to the eye surface. (The normal lid pressure = 2.5 atmospheres pressure.)

7   The flexible lens – definition.

Any lens which can be flexed when on the eye but has the properties of a hard lens.
   Example: a very thin hard lens under stress of lid pressure can become flexed.
   Flexual ability = number of times a lens is flexed to produce breakage.

8   Hysteresis.
A lens subjected to stress changes its form. When the stress is removed the lens, especially if soft, will not necessarily return to its original form. The graph shows how a contact lens material changes as stress is applied and then released.

8

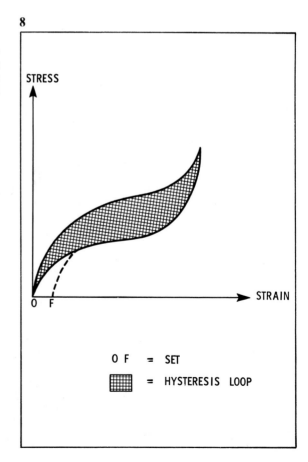

STRESS

STRAIN

O F

O F   =   SET

=   HYSTERESIS LOOP

Measurement of soft lens thickness

9 **Pachometer (pachymeter).** Using a wet cell attached to a slit-lamp a split-beam pachometer can be used. The same equipment can be used to measure a contact lens on the eye.

10 **Thickness gauge.** The conventional thickness gauge with round anvils can be wired to give a signal when the lens and the anvils make contact, so giving a reading without indenting the material. (Only for hydrophilic materials or materials with electrical conductivity.)

9

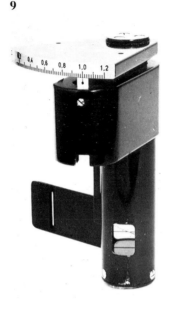

10

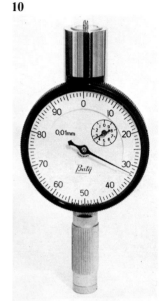

Material gas permeability (O_2) and lens permeability

11 **The gas flow through a lens** can be measured using a double chamber, the gas tensions on each side of the lens being estimated in a time period study. The solution used is N saline. Estimations at different temperatures and at different gas tension gradients can be made and given in a relative form.

11

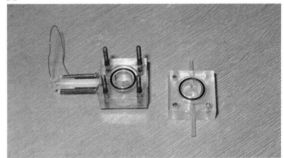

12 & 13 **The gas (O_2) tension** can be measured in the polyethylene membrane held on a polarographic (platinum) probe. This probe being held on a hydrophilic soft lens can give a time period study of the membrane uptake or degradation of oxygen tension. The probe can be held on the cornea and on the soft lens *in situ* (I. Fatt).

12

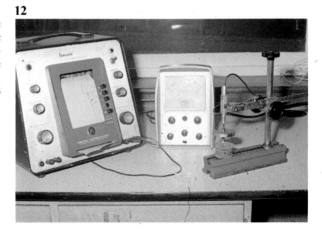

13

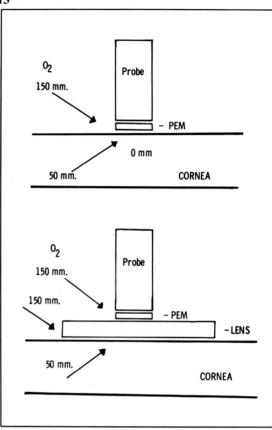

O_2 permeability = oxygen diffusion coefficient (D) × solubility of oxygen in material (k)

$= Dk \times 10^{-11}$ $(cm^2/s)(mlO_2/ml \times mm\ Hg)$

for a contact lens of thickness L

O_2 transmissibility $= \dfrac{Dk}{L} \times 10^{-9}$

14

14 Polariser. The analysis of polarised light transmitted by a material or lens will illustrate areas of material non-homogenicity. These patterns are noticed when polymers are rapidly annealed or subjected to abnormal stress.

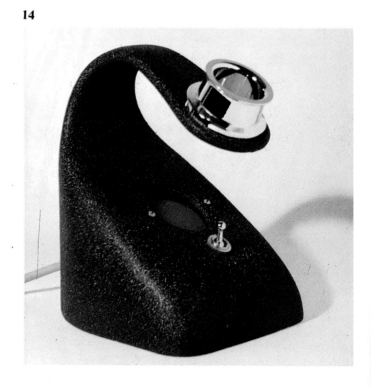

15 Material stress patterns in plastic buttons. Stress lines show in one material only, the other being the better for contact lens manufacture.

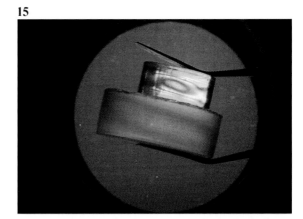

16 Material stress patterns. Another example of stress in plastic materials used in contact lens manufacture. Creep tests record the change in lens form with stress, i.e. deformation test (tensile modules).

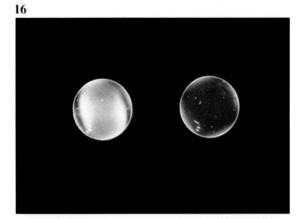

17 Micro-penetration hardness test (1). A force is applied which will penetrate the needle to a fixed distance in the lens substance. The relative hardness of lenses can be found.

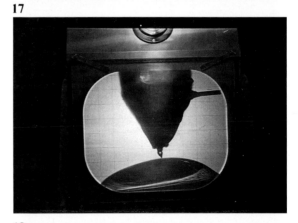

18 Micro-penetration hardness test (2). The needle is now in the lens.
   Example of results:
$$\frac{PMMA \text{ (hard lens)}}{PHEMA \text{ (soft lens) } 38\%} = \frac{50}{1}$$
The soft lens has a surface penetration one fiftieth of the hard material. Hardness = resistance to penetration. Other measurements of importance for resistance are, tensile strength, notch strength.

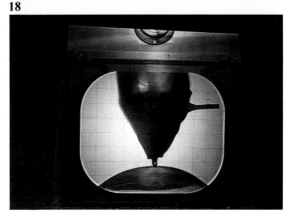

Measurement of soft lens form – shadowgraphs

19

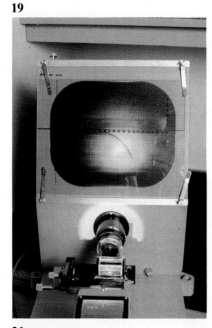

20

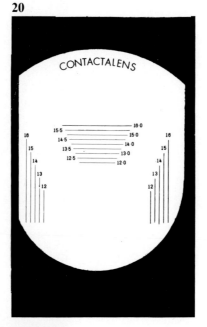

21

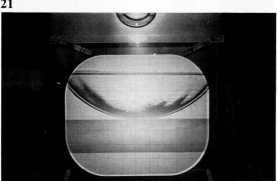

19–21 A shadowgraph when analysed will give measurements from a magnified lens profile. Whilst tolerances are limited, soft lens curvatures can be computed from chords and sagitta. The lens thicknesses can also be found by this method. The measurement can be done at 21°C as required for standard tolerances but the change in form at 33°C gives information for assessing behaviour on the eye and calculating lens temperature coefficients. Sagitta, thickness, size and curvatures can be measured by this method. (See Fig. 9 and 10 for alternative thickness method.)

22

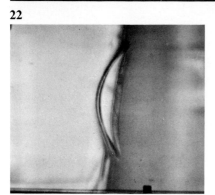

23

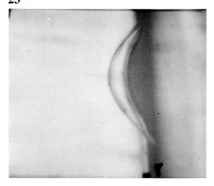

22 Shadowgraph of soft bifocal form. Solid concentric soft bifocal (Focus Laboratory). The shadowgraph illustrates the bifocal vision lens form. The outer position of the lens shown has a more positive lens power than the centre.

23 Solid concentric soft bifocal (Focus Laboratory). The shadowgraph shows the flat back curve of the small central optic zone as compared with the large near correction of the remainder of the lens. (Compare hard lens bifocal Fig. 89–93.)

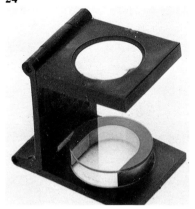

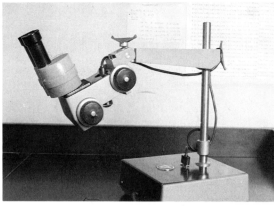

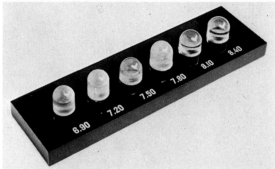

24 Simple graticule magnifier. Simple linen magnifier used to see gross flaws and also to measure size of lenses. ('V' slot diameter gauge is another method but is not illustrated.)

25 Low power binocular microscope. The instrument is used with oblique illumination for contact lens manipulations and quality control examination.

26 Spherical test domes. Set of spherical domes on which soft lenses can be placed to estimate approximate back curve.

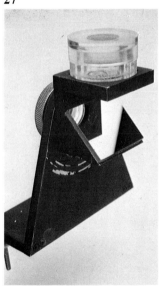

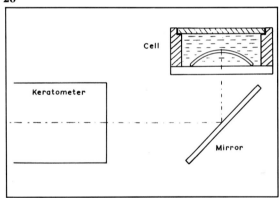

Cell

Keratometer

Mirror

27 & 28 Wet tank keratometer attachment. A tank mirror device (Chaston) to measure curves of gel contact lens using a keratometer.

29

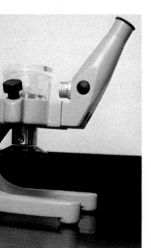

30

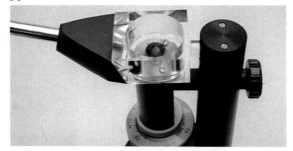

29 Wet tank sagittometer for gel lenses. A central probe is elevated to touch back apex of lens. The point of contact is sighted by an optical system. The distance from base to contact gives the sagitta. This is converted to radius measurement (see Figs. 72 and 73).

30 Sagittometer water cell (C.L.M.). Lens is coloured for demonstration.

31

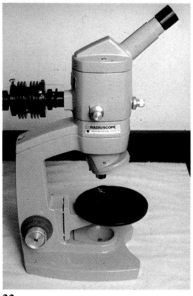

32

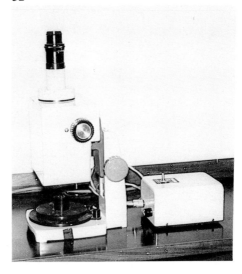

31 Radiuscope (Drysdale's principle). This instrument can be used also to measure peripheral curves and thickness of a lens. It can be coupled with an electrical digital readout (Nissel).

32 Toposcope. Using interoferometry and Moire fringes the overall curvature of a lens can be measured.

33

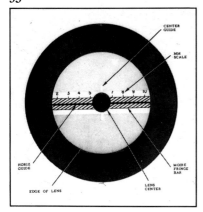

34

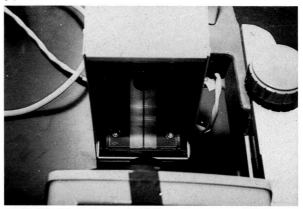

33 & 34 The alignment of the fringes over different chords gives useful information of the change in back surface curvature.

Manufacturing procedures

This section gives basic principles applicable to small laboratory work. Mass production of contact lenses uses automated lathes and polishing machines. The moulding method is especially applicable to mass production of contact lenses and good reproducibility.

The scleral (haptic) lens

35 & 36 The tray (fenestrated) is filled with special alginate and placed on the eye which has previously been anaesthetised. Using a large sucker the shell and 'set' alginate are removed.

37 Plaster is poured into the alginate shape in the tray thus making a plaster model of the eye surface.

38 An injection tray method of making the plaster eye model (on left). In the centre, a shell of polymethyl methacrylate made from the plaster model.

39 Shadowgraph of the model. A plaster model of the eye on a shadowgraph screen. The outline can be the basis of geometric lathe cut scleral lenses.

35

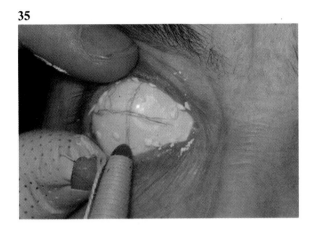

36

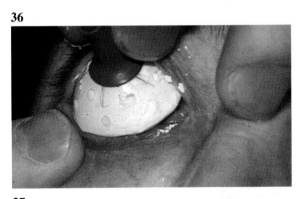

37

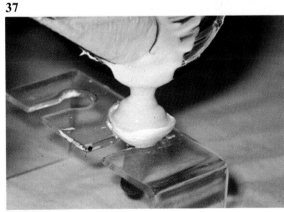

38

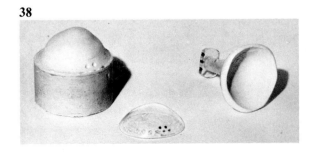

39

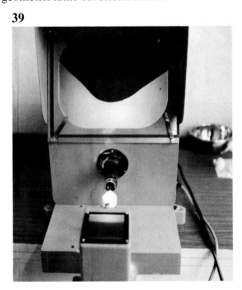

40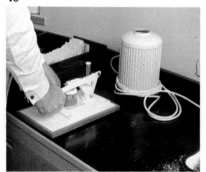

41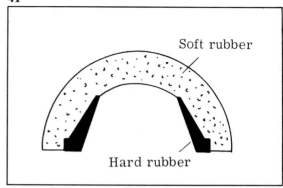

Soft rubber

Hard rubber

40 Pressing of plastic shape. A heated sheet of plastic (0.6mm thick) placed over the plaster model and a toggle pressure machine being used to form the shell shape.

41 Hand press. Cross-section of rubber or plastic ball which clamps down on to the hot sheet plastic. Note that the outer coat is soft, and the inner hard heat-resistant plastic.

42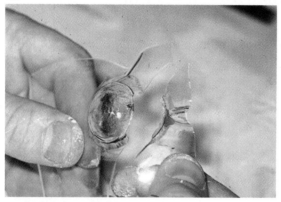

43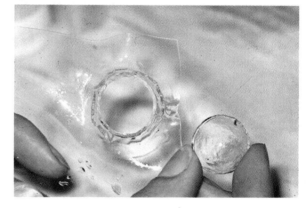

44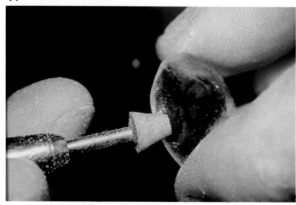

42 Plastic cooled shape. The sheet of plastic after pressing out showing the scleral shell shape.

43 Cut out of scleral shell. The shell shape cut out of the sheet.

44 Edge cutting. The edge being trimmed to correct size.

45 Edge polishing. The edge being buffed and polished.

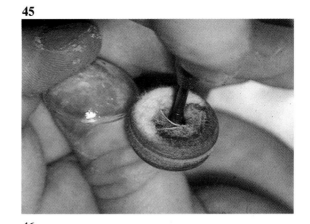

46 Fenestration (ventilation). A hole being drilled in the limbal (transition) region of the scleral lens.

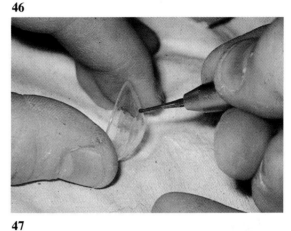

47 Tools for lapping. Two spherical diamond bonded tools which are used to lap the back optical portion of the lens.
N.B. The first optic will be cut in a lathe in the same manner as a corneal lens (see Fig. 56).

48 Bench lay-out. A lay-out on a bench to show hand drill, beeswax and several tools.

49 Vertical spindle motor. A table fitted with a vertical motorised spindle, various tools for making the back optic surface transitions, etc. Also shown is a focimeter, engraving machine and thickness gauge.

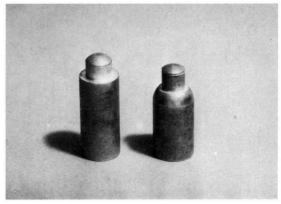

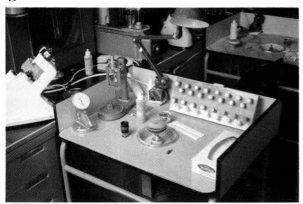

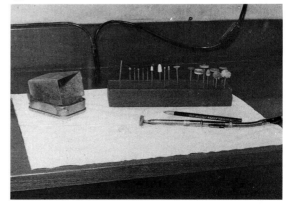

50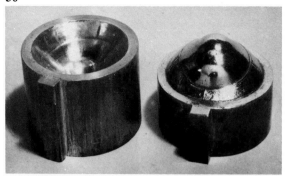

51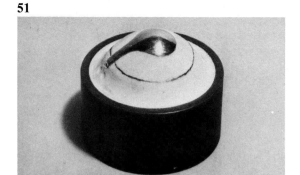

50 Positive and negative moulding tools. For production moulding work, metal female and male dye tools are prepared. Such work is done in controlled temperatures in an electric oven (150–170°C).

51 Preformed controlled clearances. An example of lamination clearances using the modified model. Preformed clearances for the shell are obtained by using metal or plastic set into the plaster. In this example a back optic combined with the channel is set on to the cast of the model.

52

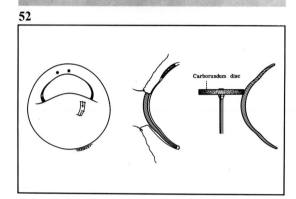

52 Slit ventilation. A scleral lens with a large slot (or slit) cut out above for ventilation or to hold up a ptosed lid (see Figs. 289–300). Trodd type. This slit principle can be used instead of fenestrations.

Corneal and intermediate hard lenses

53 Trial fitting sets for hard or rigid material lenses (including gas permeable).

Purpose	BCOR	BCOD	TD	AEL	Tc		Te	Notes
Low minus or plus Small corneal lenses −10.00−+10.00	} 7.00−8.50	7.00−8.30	7.00−8.70	0.13−0.13	minus plus	0.10 0.25	0.16 0.16	
Conventional corneal minus and plus −20.0−+20.0	7.00−8.70	7.00−8.00	9.00−10.30	0.15−0.25	high minus plus	0.08 0.25	0.18 0.18	Reduced optics for high powers
Keratoconus −4.00	5.5−7.50	6.00−7.00	9.00−9.70	0.15−0.15		0.12	0.18	Reduced optics for high powers
Intermediate (for graft or aphakic eyes) Plano or +14.00	7.80−9.00	8.00−8.40	12.00−13.00	0.25−0.35	0.10 for minus 0.45 for plus		0.20	Reduced optics for all powers Fenestrate 4 holes in intermediate area
Toric hard (truncated 1½△ base down) −4.00S −1.00−2.0−3.0 cyls	0.5 1.0 1.5mm difference in meridians	variable	9.50 9.50	0.15 0.15				

BCOR, back central optic radius; BCOD, back central optic diameter; TD, total diameter; AEL, axial edge lift; *Tc* and *Te*, centre and edge thickness.

54 Family of curves used in contact lens practice.
They are: spherical

        ellipsoidal
        paraboloidal } true asphericals

Note that hyperboloidal is rarely used.
  Pseudo-asphericals include:
    multi-spherical blended surfaces
    central spherical plus offset spherical
              plus tangent (conoids)

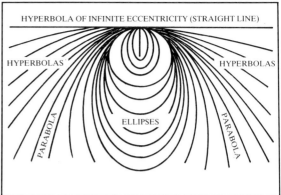

55 Plastic buttons. Button of coloured plastic for corneal lens manufacture.

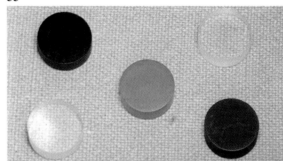

56 The lathe. Example of a lathe cutting machine (Robertson). This type of machine cuts front and back surfaces to high tolerances of accuracy and can be automated and coupled to computer control for mass production.

57 The diamond tool. The diamond tool of a lathe regressing front surface that has just been cut (Nissel lathe).

58 Dry PHEMA surface after lathe cutting. A surface of PHEMA dry plastic after diamond tool lathe cutting and before polishing – when hydrated a non-polished lens can still have a good optic.
N.B. This surface cannot be tolerated.

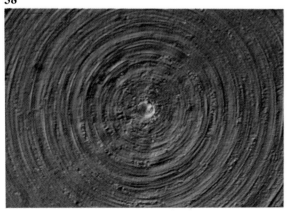

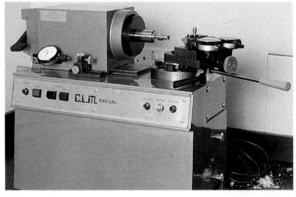

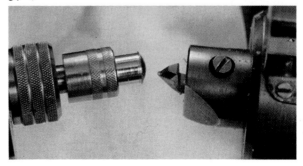

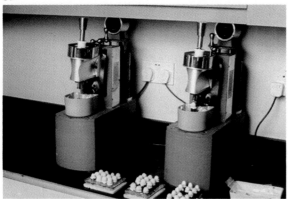

59 Surface polishing machine. A pair of polishing machines in action. Machines to make special lenses are not shown, e.g. spun moulded and torics. (See M. Ruben *Textbook of Contact Lens* (1975) Bailliere Tindall, London. See also *Soft Lenses* (1978) ed. M. Ruben, Bailliere Tindall, London and J. Wiley Inc., New York.)

60   **61**

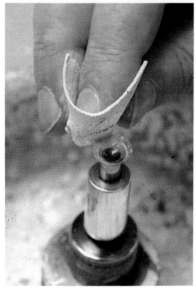 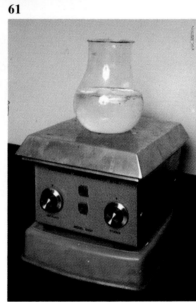

60 Hand polishing a lens edge. Automated procedures are used but many manufacturers still use hand finishing methods.

61 Hot plate vibrator. Hot plate and vibrator combined to wash out dirt and polishes from newly manufactured hard lenses.

62

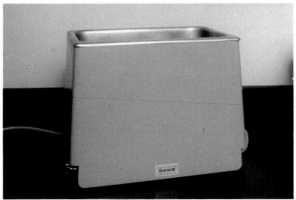

62 Ultrasonic tank. A method which removes debris from lenses by high frequency waves. The solution can be balanced saline for hydrophilic lenses. Paraffin is sometimes used for PMMA lenses.

2. Fitting procedures

General

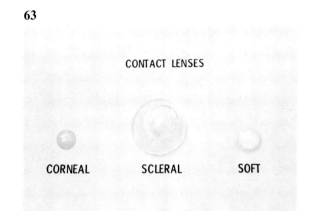

63

63 **The three chief types of lenses:** scleral (haptic) hard, corneal hard and hydrophilic soft.

N.B. Gas permeable hard lenses, because they tend to be in the size range 9–10.5mm, should be fitted flat to the average keratometry. In general the same rules as apply to all hard lenses.

---

64 Lens specifications

Types	*Total diameter*
Corneal	7.0–11.5mm
Corneo scleral	11.5–15.00mm
Scleral	16–26mm (usually vertical diameter is 1 to 3mm less than horizontal) thus $\dfrac{20V}{24H}$ Periphery (haptic) can be moulded to conform to eye shape.

Specifications of back surface	Back surface fitting curves: one or more curves or continuous (aspheric) curves.
Front surface as determined by optical power	Front surface of one or more curves, the central having a determining optical function.
	Reduced front optic when necessary to produce tolerable thicknesses.
	Central thickness (Tc) and other thickness where specified. For small diameter lenses specify Tc in minus powers.
Additional features	Fenestrations. Channels. Slots.
Material	Hard or soft (chemical type) and coated surfaces where applicable.
Solutions used with lens	As specified by manufacturer.
Methods of cleaning and disinfection	As specified by manufacturer.
Tints and colours	Homogeneous tints (transparent). Opaque tints, paintings, or photographic laminates.

65 The law of lens back surface fitting. In general the lens back surface is flatter then the eye shape. Whilst areas especially central may be in parallel or steeper than the eye shape, the peripheral surfaces must be flatter. This law applies to all contact lenses so as to prevent occlusion of the eye tissues.

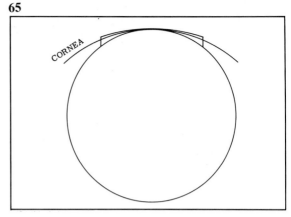

66 Choice of surface contours. The dotted line is the eye shape. On the right (CF) an aspheric is compared with spherical type curves (ABC). Such curves are spherical over central zone of 2–4mm (within practical accepted tolerances of measurement of sphericity).

The left side shows how two spherical curves with centres along the same axis can closely simulate the eye shape. The general principle of using fitting back curves, either spherical or aspherical, depends upon the size and method of lens manufacture.

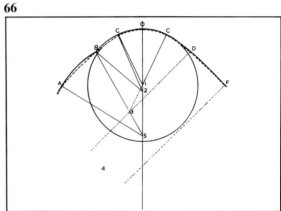

67 Best lens optical forms and contact lenses. Spectacle lens form compared with contact lens form.

With spectacle lens form the paraxial aberrations can be corrected by changing the peripheral lens curves. The periphery of a contact lens is determined largely by fitting and lens thickness and not 'best form' of lens.

The back surface influence on lens form is on average two-thirds less than on a spectacle lens form because of refractive index difference between lens and tear film.

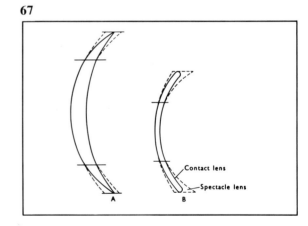

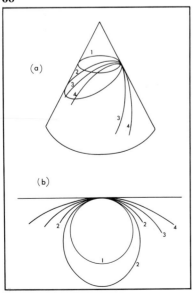

68 Curves of the cone section (conoid curves). A cone when sectioned (a) produces a circle when parallel to base. Oblique sections produce curves varying from flat ellipses to paraboloids and then hyperboloids. (b) Almost all contact lens back curves can be contained in the elliptical curves.

N.B. The corneal surface conforms essentially to a tilted ellipsoid.

Pseudo-conic surfaces

Progressive changing curves from ellipse to paraboloid obey a mathematical progression. But a combination of central spherical curves with peripheral cone or offset surfaces closely simulate true continuous curved surfaces. Figs. 69–71 are examples.

69   **70**   **71**

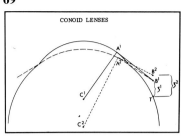

69 Central spherical and peripheral tangent. The centre is spherical and the periphery conoidal. C^2A^2 = radius of cornea.

N.B. This type of back surface is fitted centrally steeper than the cornea and over a small chord (e.g. 5.5 to 6.5) and the peripheral edge of cone designed to clear the adjacent cornea.

Many formulations are possible.

C^1A^1 steep fit C^2A^2 alignment fit
A^1B^1 tangent $3^2 > 3^1 (B^2T > B^1T)$
A^2B^2 tangent
- - - - cornea

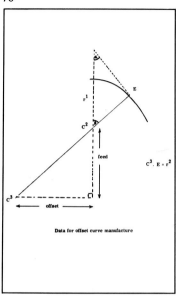

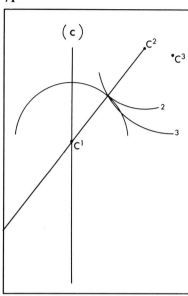

70 Central spherical and peripheral offset spherical. The centre is spherical and only slightly steeper than average keratometry. The peripheral curve has a centre off central axis C^3 and produces a continuous curve with the central. The central chord is small and this back surface is particularly useful for keratoconus cornea.

71 Pseudo-aspheric design. Can also be used for peripheral front surfaces (see soft lens).

72   **73**

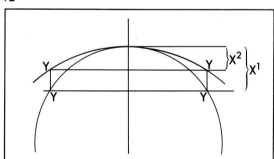

72 Specification of curves by sagitta (X in diagram):

$$r = \frac{Y^2}{2X} + \frac{X}{2}$$

$$X = r - \sqrt{r^2 - Y^2}$$

Thus any curved surface can be related to radius chords and sagitta and a conoid surface in section can so be related. Every contact lens has an overall or total sagitta and given the central back spherical curve and its chord, the peripheral form can then be designed if the *overall* or total sagitta is known.

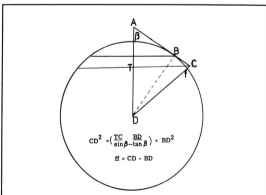

$$CD^2 = \left(\frac{TC}{\sin\beta} \cdot \frac{BD}{\tan\beta} \right) + BD^2$$

$$ff = CD - BD$$

73 Axial edge lift (AEL) (3)–(or $\int\!\int$). The distance from the edge of a lens to the back central curve can be measured radially or perpendicularly (radially in diagram). Given the central back radius and chord, the total diameter and the axial edge lift, the back surface of a lens can be designed.

N.B. The corneal surface is approximately mid-point between the extension of the central curve and the edge of the lens, *see* Fig. **65**.

74 & 75 Derivation of equations for conic sections (A. G. Bennett).

$$P = \text{eccentricity factor} = \frac{2r_0X - Y^2}{X^2}$$

$$\text{(eccentricity)} \quad E = \frac{1 - 2r_0(X^2 + 3) - Y^2}{(X^2 + 3)^2}$$

$$P = 1 - E^2$$
$$\text{parabola} \quad = Y = AX^2$$
$$= Y^2 = 2f(1+E)X - (1-E^2)X^2$$

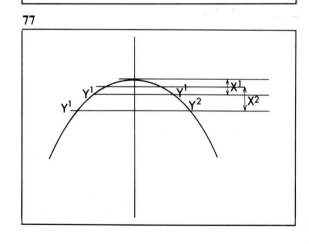

Derivation of the equation to a conic section when the origin of co-ordinates is placed at the vertex of the curve.

75

More about 'P'. The P value or degrees of curvature eccentricity are related in this graph to the 3 values for different apertures (diameter of lens). As the eccentricity increases and the diameter of the lens likewise so will the (axial edge lift) increase.

N.B. Large lens design (over 9mm size) must use peripheral curves with fine tolerances because of the total eccentricity changes induced.

P values above 0 to 0.80
A.E.L. below 0 to 0.25
Size 6 to 10mm

76 Junction of spherical and toric surfaces. Back surface of central spherical with peripheral toric surfaces. The central surface has an oval outline. It is possible to decentre the spherical zone relative to the peripheral toric.

77 Sagitta and continuous curves. In this diagram the sagitta are designated as X since they are in the X coordinate, Y symbols are in the opposite coordinate and refer to the chords. Thus the upper aspheric curve is related to the circle (or back central optic zone) over a small chord which is not labelled and in practice is only 2–4mm. The axial edge lift is $X^1 - X^2$ (cf. Fig. 72).

P VALUES
(eccentricity quotient)

0.8   0.6   0.4   0.2   0

APERTURES IN MM.

0   0.05   0.10   0.15   0.20   0.25

3 VALUES

Bennett's '3' values given for different overall diameters 6 to 10 mm, for contours having different eccentricity values.

76

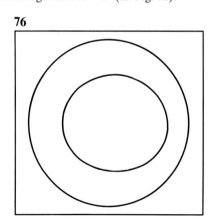

77

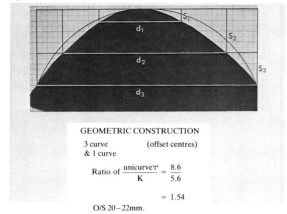

GEOMETRIC CONSTRUCTION

3 curve   (offset centres)
& 1 curve

$$\text{Ratio of } \frac{\text{unicurve 'r'}}{K} = \frac{8.6}{5.6}$$

$$= 1.54$$

O/S 20 – 22mm.

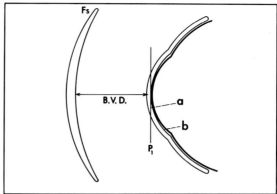

78 Large lens construction from eye mould. The projection of the eye shape can form the basis of sagitta measurement and then a lens form can be designed. Using chords less than 8mm (of the eye) will lead to gross errors by this technique. Soft or hard material can be lathe cut to these designs.

79 Power of a contact lens. This can be calculated as the ocular refraction if the back surface of the contact lens is the same as the cornea over a 6mm chord (approx).

$$\text{contact lens} = Fs/(1 - dFs)$$

Allowances must be made if the back curve is different to the average keratometry K (0.5D for each 0.1mm difference in radius of curvature, + for steeper and − for flatter than K.

(Fs = spectacle refraction)
(d = BVD back vertex distance.)

80 Testing for correct power of contact lens. A trial contact lens can be used and the spectacle overcorrection (OC) added to the power of the contact lens.

N.B. Effective power calculation necessary if spectacle correction is over ± 5.0D.

81 Transition of surfaces. The junction of two different curved surfaces is often blended in practice to form a transition. This smoothing process is necessary to avoid trauma. Therefore chord size is very difficult to measure in the finished lens.

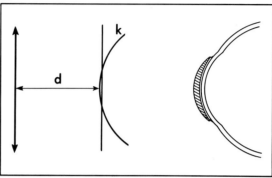

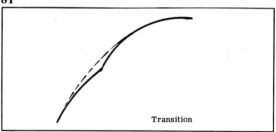

Transition

Stabilisation of contact lenses

1. Normal centration by at least three zones of contact, e.g. central and two peripheral or three peripheral or two back peripheral and upper lid front contact (see Fig. 101).
2. Other methods of stabilisation:
   Back surface aspheric curves
   Truncations
   Ballasting (prism base down)
   Palpebral peripheral thickness increase (Fig. 125)
   Toric lens.

83

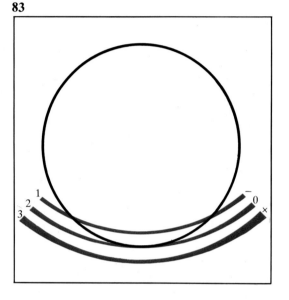

83 Lid position and truncations. This is determined by size of lens relative to position of lower lid and limbus. Diagram shows three positions of lower lid in primary position of gaze.

1, above limbus	−
2, at limbus	0
3, below limbus (scleral gap)	+

84 Truncation insets. For corneal lenses covering two-thirds of corneal surface, the following is advised.

	Lower lid position	Truncation
1	−	1mm inset
2	0	0.5mm inset
3	+	no truncation

85 Prism ballast.

	Powers	
	0 − −8.0	−8.0 and over
For negative lenses	$1^\triangle$	$1.5^\triangle$
For plus lenses use negative peripheral optics carrier	$2^\triangle$	$2^\triangle$

The prism ballast is often combined with a truncation. Plus lens stabilisation is a difficult fitting to achieve.

Bifocal hard lens designs

Several designs are available. Concentric and continuous curves (both solid forms) and segment fused forms are the types most commonly used.

86   Concentric central distance fused with peripheral materials of different refractive indices.

87   Concentric back curve bifocal.

88   Central distance with peripheral near – solid form. In this form a small back optic zone is used for distance. The front curve is single.
   Example: Back surface

		Radii	Diameters
1	BCOR	8.40	5.00
2		8.00	9.60
3		12.00	9.80

Front optic radius = 8.30.. Centre portion = −4.50 Sphere. Near portion = −2.50 Sphere.
   The above figures are illustrative only and based on refractive index 1.50. It assumes that the 8.00 back curve will give a flat fitting for the large size of lens (9.8) and also that the central back of 0.40 flatter than peripheral will produce a functional power of −4.50. In this example the average K was 7.60.

89   Truncated fused segment hard corneal bifocal lens. The fitting must take into account the position of the segment below centre and the position of the lower lid (see Fig. 84). The width of near segment is therefore often limited.

86

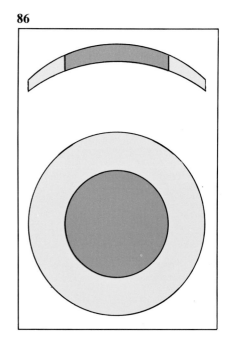

87

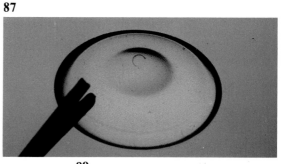

88

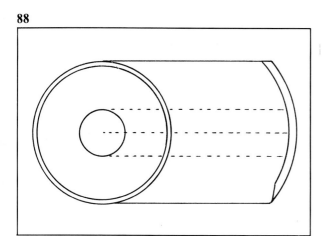

89

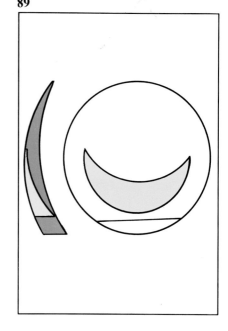

90 & 91 Mode of operation. In the reading position of the eye the near point of the near segment should be in the line of vision. Thus if a patient with the eyes in the primary position is seen to have a lower edge of lid 1mm above the limbus, a truncation of 1mm will place the geometric centre of a 10mm lens in the optical axis of the distance portions. A further depression of gaze of only a few degrees would bring the near point into the visual line. OA is the visual line and Fig. 90 shows the position of the lens in the primary position of the eye. Fig. 91 shows the eye in the reading position, the dotted line being the visual line for the first eye position.

90

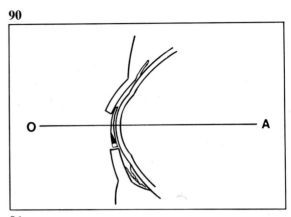

91

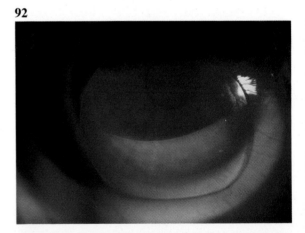

92 Fused segment bifocal. Truncated segmented bifocal corneal hard lens. Note position of top of segment.

92

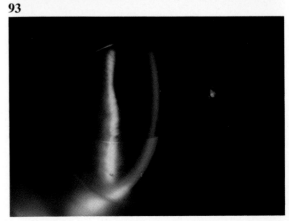

93 Fused segment bifocal on the eye. Some near sequents (of higher refractive index) fluoresce and assist fitting.

93

Fitting of hard corneal lenses

Principles.
1. Centration with corneal ventilation.
2. Minimal movement on versions of eye.
3. Lid tolerance and lens control with blinking permitting vertical excursions of the lens.

94   Insertion of lens. Some patients can insert without upper lid retraction. Removal is by breaking the surface tension adhesion between lens and cornea. The eye is depressed whilst upper or lower edge of lens is gently pressed against eye by tightening the lids with finger pressure.

94

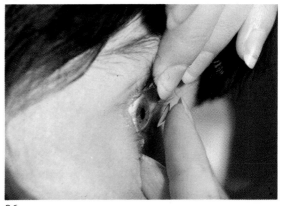

95

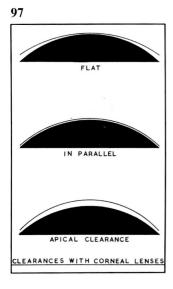

96

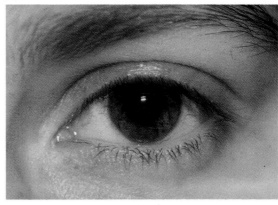

95 & 96   Myopia. Right and left eyes, both fitted with the following back curve lenses:

$$\text{radii} \left\{ \begin{array}{l} 7.90 : 7.70 \\ 9.00 : 8.50 \\ 11.50 : 8.75 \end{array} \right\} \text{diam.}$$

$Tc = 0.10$, $Te = 0.16$, average $K = 7.60$.

N.B. The right lid is lower than left. This lens-induced ptosis is due to poor edge design (faulty manufacture showed right edge $t = 0.25$ compared with left edge $t = 0.20$). The right upper lid had oedema (Fig. 95).

97   The basic fits.
  Overall flat fit.
  Parallel fit.
  Central clearance with peripheral touch, the central clearance being minimal (approx. 0.06mm depth).

98   Diagram of parallel fit. Only an aspheric back surface can give a parallel fit. But in practice a single spherical surface produces a clinically acceptable parallel fit for small diameter and a multi-spherical back curve for large diameters.

97

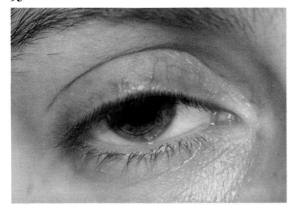

FLAT

IN PARALLEL

APICAL CLEARANCE

CLEARANCES WITH CORNEAL LENSES

98

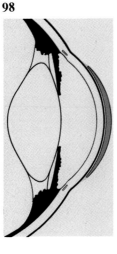

37

Assessment of fit

To assess fit use the following methods.
White light with magnification of × 2:
note centration with eye movement of gaze,
note centration with convergence for near fixation,
note centration with blinking.
Blue light with fluorescein – note as for white light.
Slit-beam microscope – note zones of tissue touch and
compression of vessels (conjunctival).

99 Fit diagrams. *Left* shows overall parallel fit with
peripheral edge clearance. *Right* shows central
clearance, intermediate contact peripheral back edge
clearance.

100 Fluorescein patterns of fit – parallel fit. Section of a
9.30mm hard gas permeable lens (MO_2) to show almost
parallel fit (courtesy of Menicon).

101 Fluorescein pattern of central parallel fit. Diagram
shows central minimal touch and peripheral contact.
Arrows indicate fluid movement. All fittings whilst
assessed in primary position *must* be considered with eye
movement, i.e. the lens fitting is DYNAMIC not static.

102 Upper lid and contact lens fit. Diagrams show
central clearance (steep fit) and prismoid edge clearance
below (flat fit). The lens can be made to move with the
upper lid by adhesion if the edge has negative form. This
results in decentration when upper lid retraction occurs.

103 Parallel central fit. Whilst the central fit is parallel
the edge fitting shows excessive clearance especially in
eye movement.

Prismoid Inferior Clearance	Central Clearance
	Intermediate and Peripheral Contact
	Edge Meniscus

102

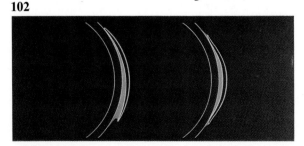

Parallel fit | Central Clearance
Peripheral Zone Contact
Edge Lift

99 Right   Left

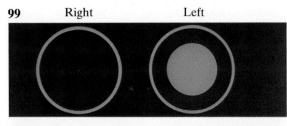

100

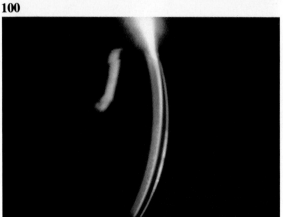

101

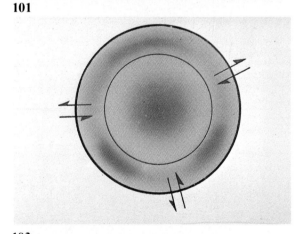

103

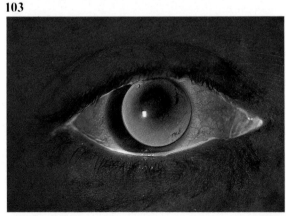

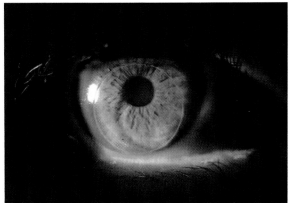

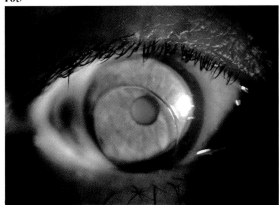

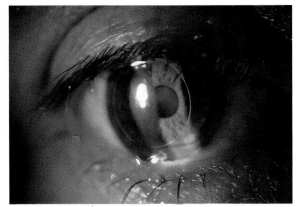

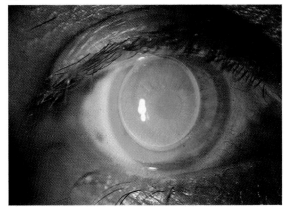

104–107 A small lens negative power fittings. Figs. 104–107 show good centration between blinking, but without lid movement the lens sags downwards. Many low myopes tolerate this fitting very well.

Back curve for small lens design is:

$$BCOR = 0.2 + AV.\ K$$
$$T.D. = 0.2 + AV.\ K$$

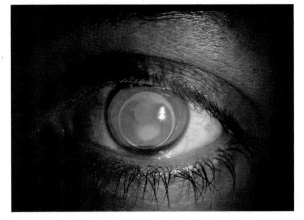

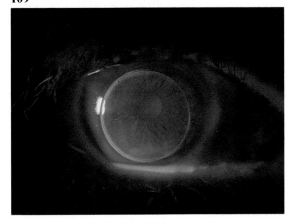

108–110 A small (inter-palpebral fitting). Diameter (7.9mm) corneal hard lens to show parallel fitting and edge clearance.

The back curve is single curve except for the peripheral edge lift.

Example: Av. $k.$ = 7.7mm. Back curve: 7.90 : 7.70/ 10.50 : 7.90. P = −4.00 Tc = 0.10
Te = 0.16

These lenses must be thin with perfect edge finish. For positive powers central thickness must not exceed 0.25mm. Best to fit this lens on steep cornea with

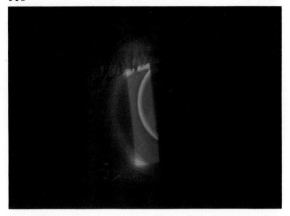

palpebral fissures of vertical size 10–12mm. Gas permeable materials of low CAB and silicone and low water content only possible for this lens form.

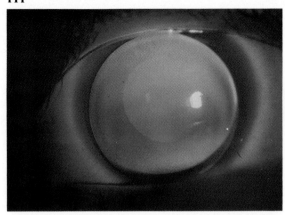

111 Menicon MO$_2$ fitting – a gas permeable lens with surface having hydrophilic properties (Figs. 111–113). The photograph is of a normal flatter than *K* fitting for a 9.3mm total diameter size lens.

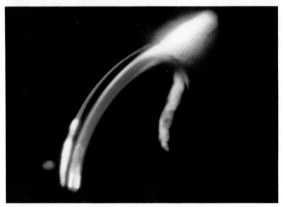

112 A section to show too loose edge fitting.

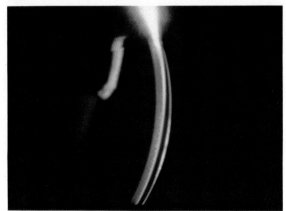

113 A section to show satisfactory edge fitting.

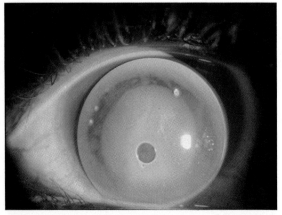

114 A section to show tight edge fitting. This fitting is not satisfactory since there is also excessive central clearance which will lead to occlusion oedema.

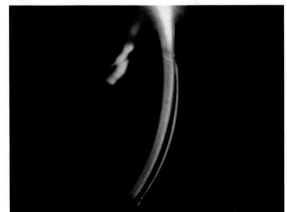

115 Central corneal clearance. Minimal central clearance is acceptable.

116 Large corneal lenses and excessive clearance centrally with locked bubble. Both fits are of doubtful acceptance unless a central fenestration is used (e.g. in aphakia). This type of fitting using gas permeable hard materials should be avoided.

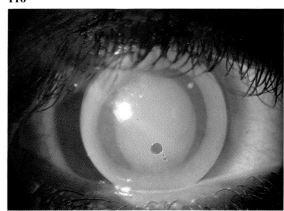
116

Toroidal hard lenses

Chief types:
    toroidal front optic,
    toroidal back surface (central and peripheral),
    toroidal peripheral back surface with central spherical.

117 Toroidal fluid lens. Back surface toric. Indications: to stabilise and centre a lens on astigmatic cornea; to introduce astigmatic corrections; to produce better tear lens exchange (peripheral torics).

    Diagram shows central toroid form of the tear lens. This surface will *induce* astigmatism.

N.B. Toric patterns may be due to toric forms of eye or toric forms of back surface of lens.

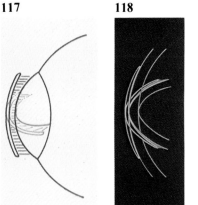
117

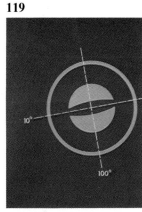
118   119

118 Toric fluorescein patterns – spherical lens back surface on toric cornea. This form will negate most of the corneal astigmatism.

N.B. Hard and thick soft forms can produce *residual* astigmatism which can be compensated by front torics.

119 Toric fluorescein patterns. Diagram of fluorescein with a toric cornea and spherical contact lens curvatures.

> Vertical – Parallel Fit
> Horizontal – Central Contact
>   Peripheral Clearance

> Toric Central Clearance in 100° axis
> Central Contact in 10°axis
> Peripheral zone contact Edge Lift

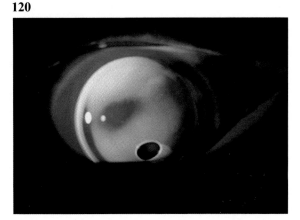
120

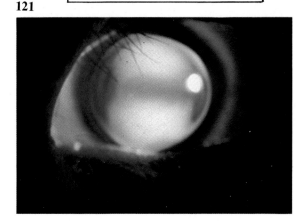
121

120 & 121 Examples of lens showing astigmatism of cornea. Zones of contact centrally indicate axis or corneal flatter curvature. Thus in Fig. 120 flatter curve was 20° and 170° for Fig. 121.

122 Astigmatic corneal fittings. Diagram of central and peripheral clearance in one axis with touch peripherally in opposite axis. This cornea is best fitted with peripheral toroidal surface.

N.B. Toric patterns may be due to toric forms of eye or toric forms of back surface of lens.

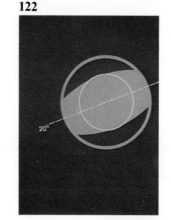

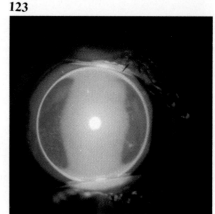

123 Astigmatic corneal fitting. Example of a spherical back curve on toric type cornea (Menicon).

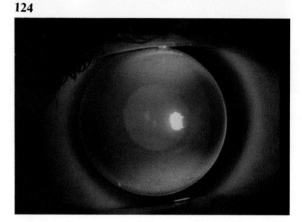

124 Toroidal peripheral back surface contact lens (on similar cornea). Example: *K* 7.40 axis 17°, 8.20 axis 80°. Average *K* 7.80.

Back curves spherical contact lens prescription: 7.40 : 7.40/9.00 : 8.50/11.50 : 8.80.

Refitted with peripheral toric and flatter central zone: 7.80 : 7.00/8.40 : 8.50 (flattest axis) 11.50 : 8.80.

$$\overline{9.20}$$

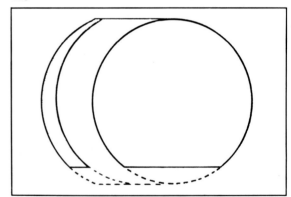

125–127 Prism ballast and truncations. Back toric surfaces of R I materials greater than R I 1.33 will induce an astigmatic effect which can be complementary to the correction of the eye's astigmatism or can be compensated by introducing a cylinder on the first surface. Wherever a cylinder is introduced on to the first surface, if the lens is not stabilised by its shape or back surface fitting, then a prism base down with or without truncation can be used (ballast). The diagrams show methods of truncating corneal hard and soft lenses, even an oval shape.

Example: Back surface at centre zone

$$\frac{7.20 \times 180°}{8.00 \times 90°} : 7.50 \text{ etc.}$$

= induced astigmatism of 4 dioptres.

Therefore the front surface must have a cyl. power equal and opposite to compensate. In practice trial back toric lenses prove very useful and the over-correction by trial spectacle lenses will, when added to the contact lens power, give the power required for the final lens.

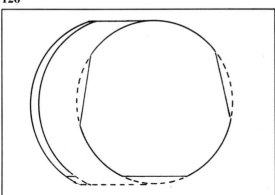

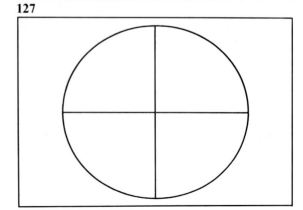

Fitting by photokeratometry – PEK (Wessley Jessen)

128

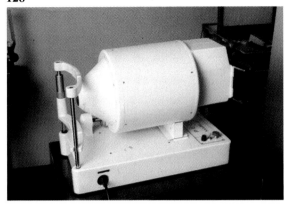

129

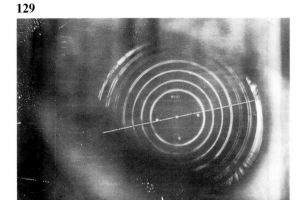

130

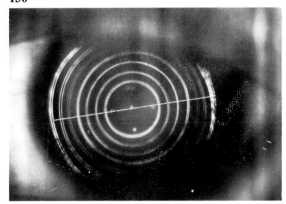

128 A simplified fitting system based on corneal image photography.

129 & 130 Photokeratometry. The corneal image photograph is analysed to give vertical and horizontal readings to form a topographical analysis of the central 10mm of cornea.

131 The coefficients of eccentricity (shape factor). Together with the power and data relating to curvature the manufacturers and practitioners feed back, a contact lens form and power is designed. The lines present the nominal shape factor and the reading; + = horizontal, ★ = vertical.

The central equivalent radius is computed. In the example shown

> Right 175° = 7.38 Right 85° = 7.37
> Left   H = 7.47   Left   V = 7.36

The hard and soft lens fitting is based upon the curves shown and an allowance of 0.015mm tear lens thickness.

Example:

Small hard lens   Right   7.41 : 8.00/11.8 : 8.1
Back curves   Left   7.51 : 8.00/12.6 : 8.1
and 26% water content (soft)

Back curves { Right   8.45/12.80
            { Left   8.70/12.80

(courtesy Wessley Jessen)

131

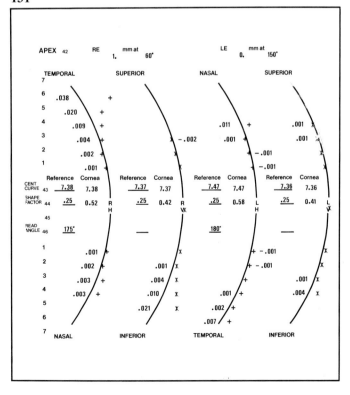

Aphakic hard lenses

132 Aphakic corneal lens correction producing bifocal effect. The aphakic lens shown is of total diameter 8.8mm but using gas permeable materials such as CAB or mixtures of CAB with silicone acrylate they can be fitted as large as 10.0mm (e.g. Boston, Polycon, Alberta, and other gas permeable materials).

To produce a near vision effect the front optic diameter must overlap the back central optic. The secondary back curve should be optical in quality and at least 1mm in width and 0.6mm flatter than the centre curve. In Fig. 132 the lens power is +16.0 and the BCOR = 7.80

$$TD = 8.50mm$$
$$Front\ optic = 7.4$$

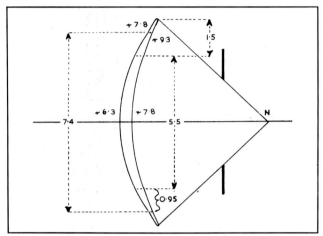

132

133 Lens on eye – corneal size. Example of 9.5mm (total diameter) aphakic lens fitted to aphakic eye. Note. minimal apical clearance and wide intermediate band.

Back curve prescription: 7.90 : 7.00/8.50 : 9.30/ 12.00 : 9.70. Front optic diameter: 8.50mm. Peripheral front curve – negative.

134 Lens on eye – intermediate size. 12.50mm CAB lathe cut lens for aphakia when conventional lenses would not centre (due to corneal apex displacement).

Back surface prescription: 8.60 : 8.20/9.00 : 12.50. Front optic diameter: 8.20mm. $Tc = 0.20$. K readings: $7.30 \times 160°$, $7.90 \times 50°$.

135 Fluorescein pattern of intermediate size eye lens (13mm) on an aphakic cornea to show areas of touch and the upward displacement of the cornea apex (diagrammatic).

133

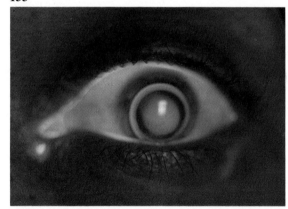

134

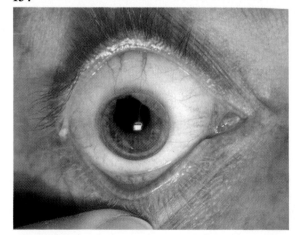

135

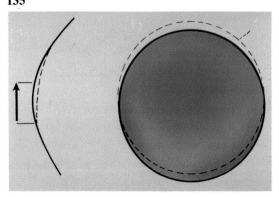

Keratoconus fitting of hard lenses

136 & 137 Variation of back central optical chord size.
C, B & D fittings (C, B & D refer to back curve design)
where C = central chord 5mm, B = central chord 6mm,
D = central chord 7mm.

Trial lenses are designed to combine variations in total
diameter with the above central chords for each central
radii.

Examples – using fenestrating at intermediate zones:
early keratoconus – central cone, B fitting, small lens
(8–9mm); early keratoconus – eccentric cone, D fitting,
large lens (9–10mm); advanced keratoconus – central
cone, C fitting, normal size (8.5–9.5mm); advanced
keratoconus – eccentric cone, C fitting, large lens
(9–10.5mm); fluorescein pattern on left = lens hanging
on cone; fluorescein pattern on right = lens hanging
from upper lid adhesion.

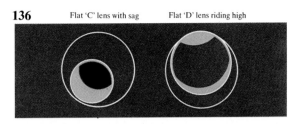

136 Flat 'C' lens with sag   Flat 'D' lens riding high

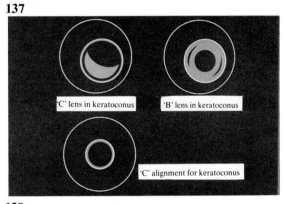

137

'C' lens in keratoconus   'B' lens in keratoconus

'C' alignment for keratoconus

138 Corneal Fleischer's ring as seen with blue light.
The size of the ring will help determine overall lens
diameter. If ring is larger than 10mm corneal fittings are
very difficult.

N.B. Ring increases in size as cone advances.

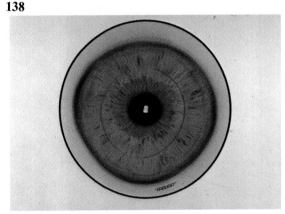

138

139 & 140 A hard corneal lens of 8.90mm diameter
with back central optic chord of 6.00mm. Note good
central stabilised fitting.

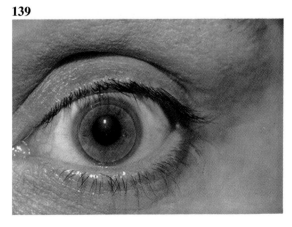

139

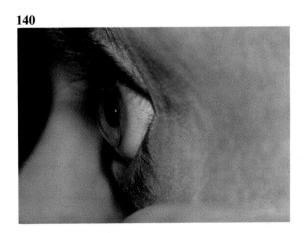

140

141, 142 & 143   An 8.70mm (Polycon material) sized lens fitted to right and left keratoconic eyes, note the left cone is steepest.

The fluorescein patterns for the right with white light and 142, 143 with blue light show cone-contact lens touch centrally with intermediate clearance. The patient preferred the left loose fitting. If corneal oedema occurs, fenestrations are advised (0.30mm diameter and 1.5mm inset).

Fluorescein pattern shows typical cone touch centrally, intermediate clearance and peripheral zones of touch but with edge clearance. If oedema of cornea occurs the lens should be fenestrated in the intermediate zone (even with gas permeable materials).

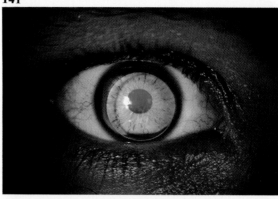

142

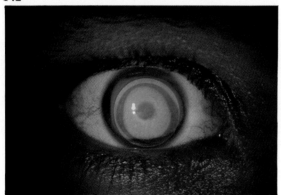

143

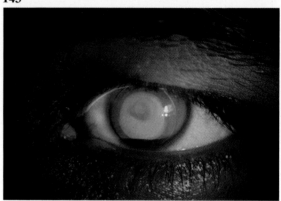

	Right eye	Left eye
K readings	6.00 irregular	5.80 irregular
Back lens surface	6.40 : 6.00	6.00 : 6.00
	7.80 : 7.00	7.60 : 7.00
	8.80 : 8.00	8.60 : 8.00
	9.00 : 8.50	8.90 : 8.50
	11.00 : 8.70	11.00 : 8.70
	Tc = 0.12	Tc = 0.09
	power = −4.00	power = −8.00
	Te = 0.16	Te = 0.16

A lens fitting – example: Corneal lens fitting for early keratoconus K 6.9 × 10° 7.20.

Back curves:	7.00 : 6.00	**Alternative fitting:**	
	8.00 : 8.60		7.00 : 6.00
	9.00 : 9.20	offset to	9.20 AEL 0.13
	11.50 : 9.50		11.50 : 9.50
	Tc = 0.12		Tc = 0.12
	Te = 0.16		Te = 0.16
	power = −6.00		power = −6.00

Two fenestrations, 0.3mm diameter, 2mm inset.

144   Small corneal apical fitting for central cone.

6.00 : 5.00	
8.00 : 6.90	
9.00 : 7.20	

Tc	=	0.08
Te	=	0.13
power	=	−10.50

N.B. This is only possible when the cone is central.

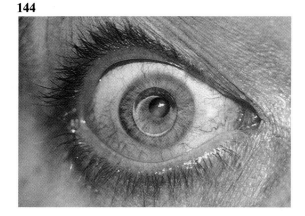

144

145   Fitting flat. Flat fitting lens for moderate cone (central).

$$K = 7.00 \rightarrow 175$$
$$6.50 \downarrow 85$$

Two positions for wear   1. sag and resting on lower lid
or,   2. held by upper lid (riding high)

Back curvature of lens: 7.20 : 6.00
offset with AEL of: 0.15 to 9.20mm
   11.00 : 9.50

N.B. Sagging of lens but well tolerated owing to relative insensitivity of cone zone.

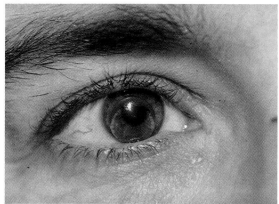

145

Keratoplasty fittings

146   Keratoplasty corneal shape. Section from mould of corneal graft, to show irregularities and small area of spherical curvature. p = 0.33 for area of graft (p = reciprocal of eccentricity squared).

147   Astigmatism and keratoplasty. To show changes in astigmatism in an 8mm penetrating graft over a period of two years. Note that astigmatism is within 15° of the 'with the rule'.

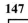

146

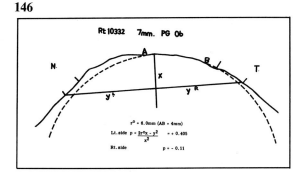

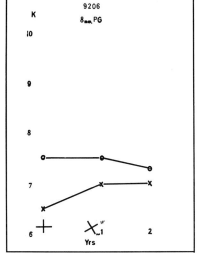

47

148 Contour of a keratoplasty. Penetrating grafts tend to have steeper than normal curvatures over small chords which are eccentric to geometric centre of cornea. Fitting of corneal hard lenses should proceed as for keratoconus.

Key: Graft shape = conoidal corneal cap.
Using same chord (BOD) a steeper curve (centre 'C') will achieve a fitting.

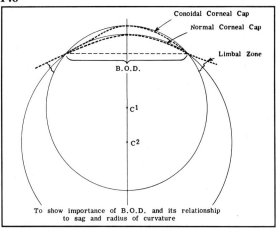

148

Conoidal Corneal Cap
Normal Corneal Cap
Limbal Zone
B.O.D.
c¹
c²

To show importance of B.O.D. and its relationship to sag and radius of curvature

149 Normal corneal and keratoplasty curves. Normal corneal curve (dotted line) is flatter than graft curve in an average.

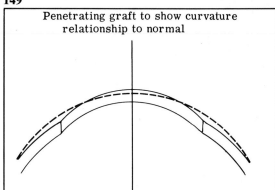

149

Penetrating graft to show curvature relationship to normal

150 Penetrating keratoplasty – corneal lenses. The corneal hard lens will nearly always bridge the graft edge – host cornea zone.

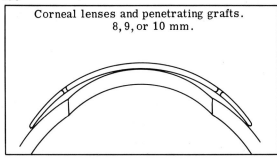

150

Corneal lenses and penetrating grafts.
8, 9, or 10 mm.

151 Corneal contact lens fitted to a penetrating graft. Note that the fitting is flatter than the corneal graft curvature which is generally advised for corneal size lenses.

152 Penetrating keratoplasty – intermediate lens. Intermediate hard lenses will produce stability and centration.

152

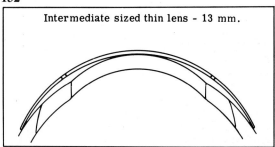

Intermediate sized thin lens - 13 mm.

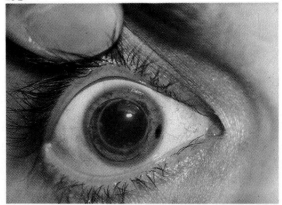

151

153 Lamellar keratoplasty. Lamellar grafts in general have flatter curves than penetrating grafts. Lamellar grafts are often larger than penetrating grafts. Therefore contact lens can be smaller than graft or larger, depending upon graft eye.

153

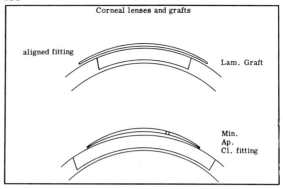

154 Intermediate size lens fitting (13mm). CAB.

Penetrating graft 8mm $K = 6.95 \times 100$
$\qquad\qquad\qquad\qquad\quad 7.40$

Lens fitting back curve: $7.90 : 8.00$
$\qquad\qquad\qquad\qquad\;\; 8.50 : 11.00$
$\qquad\qquad\qquad\qquad\;\; 9.00 : 13.00$

$Tc \;=\; 0.10$
$Te \;=\; 0.18$
power $= -4.00$. Reduced front optic: 8.50.

N.B. Central touch, peripheral touch.

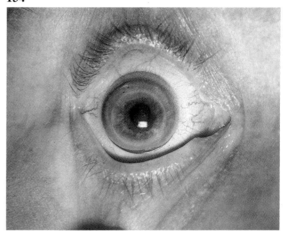

155 & 156 CAB 13mm lens. 13mm CAB hard lens on a 7mm penetrating graft, and its fluorescein pattern.

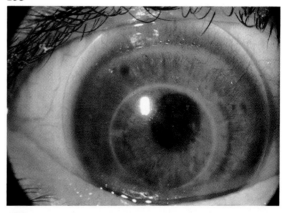

157 Fluorescein pattern and 13mm lens. Graft and CAB lens (13mm). Note the graft contact with lens.

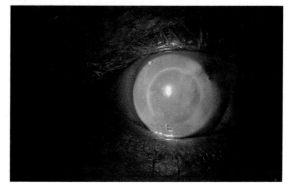

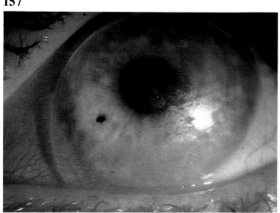

158   Fluorescein pattern of 13mm lens. Fluorescein pattern to show air bubble during extremes of movement.

N.B. Gas permeable hard lathe cut large lenses can alter curvatures and become larger and flatter as water uptake and $T°$ increases. This applies to negative lens forms. The size of air bubble and its position must be evaluated as for scleral lens fitting (*see* pages 66–69). Thus there are fenestrations over sealed areas.

158

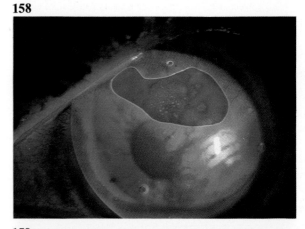

159

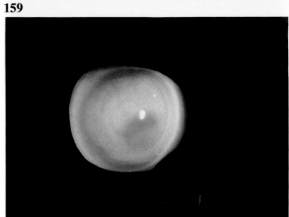

159   Fluorescein pattern of 13mm lens on a graft eye made of PMMA material.

Soft contact lens fitting

160   Soft lens: determinants of size and thickness.

Size (mm)	Fitting tolerances	Comfort	Complications
13.50–15.00	crude	good	chronic lid and corneal occlusion problems
11.50–13.50	fine	edge design determines comfort	poor edge design causes intolerance and corneal changes with flat fittings

This supposes all fittings are functional.

---

161   Thickness. This is related to volume of the lens and maximum and minimum zones. Average thickness should be known.

Power	Thickness	Optics	Complications
Plus	centre and front optic junctional thickness must be controlled	reduced optic necessary	central corneal occlusion
Negative	peripheral thickness must be controlled	reduced optic necessary	limbal occlusion

162 Water content and thickness.

Hydrophilic lenses	Thickness
High water content above 55%	av. of 0.30mm
Low water content	av. of 0.10mm

N.B. An average 0.10mm thickness would require a centre thickness of approximately 0.07mm for the following lens example 8.00/13mm, power −8.0.

163 Factors controlling centration of soft lens.

Material elasticity	Lens size
Good	small 11.75–12.50mm fitted on K or steeper very thin lenses essential
Poor	large 12.50–15.00mm fitted flatter than K

164 Areas of eye contact.
One essential difference to note is that irrespective of the geometric form a soft lens has *in vitro*, when inserted it conforms to the eye shape to a variable degree. Also there are many that have to conform to a scleral fitting, because of size or movement on to the sclera.

Relationships of areas of contact: white central area = corneal contact (12mm diam.); white and yellow central areas = corneal contact plus ½mm scleral (13mm diam.); white and yellow and orange areas = corneal plus scleral contact of 1½mm scleral (15mm diam.).

Size of soft lens	% Area of contact		Fitting radius of back surface
	With cornea	With sclera	
12	100	0	av. K + 0.40mm
13	90	10	av. K + 0.6mm
15	70	30	av. K + 1.2mm

N.B. The large lens has a scleral fitting factor that is very significant, hence a very flat back radius of curvature. Alternatively back aspheric or bicurve design is used.

This table relates only to PHEMA, Tc 0.10, e.g. power −4.00.

164b

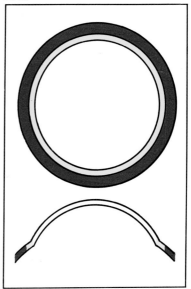

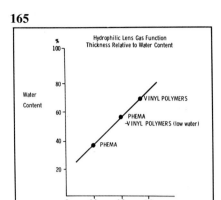

165

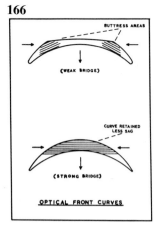

166

165 Water content and thickness. For a 28% water material lens an average thickness of under 0.10mm is necessary but for a 70% water lens 0.25mm is permissible. This is almost directly related to gas permeability.

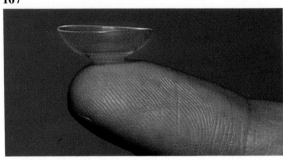

167

166 Lens bending. Material rigidity, thickness and fit, will determine wrapping of lens when on the eye. The plus lens if well centered, should give an optical surface more closely related to lens *in vitro* than a negative lens. High power lenses may show a change in power relative to degree of wrap.

167 Lens form. Soft lens held on finger. The form shown is correct and not inverted. This form for hydrophilic lenses after allowing lens to dry on finger for one minute before insertion (compare with Figs. 19–21).

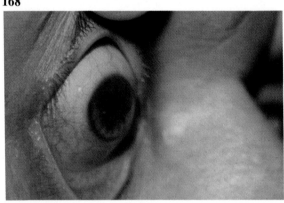

168

168 Soft lens on the eye (size 14.00mm). This lens is well centered but will move on gentle pressure and spring back to original position.

169 A well positioned hydrophilic lens of 13.50mm total diameter. This lens was 0.60mm flatter back curve than average keratometry.

170 Sagging. Soft lens (hydrophilic) 10 minutes after insertion – note sagging downwards.

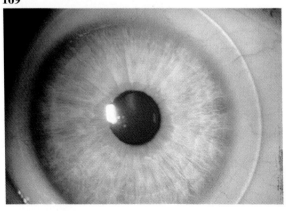

169

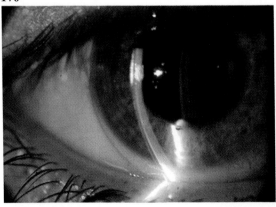

170

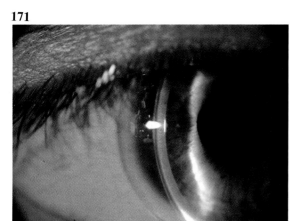

171 Centration of lens. Soft lens (hydrophilic) 30 minutes after insertion. Note centration now accurate.

172 Steep fitting of lens. Soft lens (hydrophilic) immediately upon insertion with bubble trapped and suggesting too steep a fit.

173 Steep fit and PEK image. Steep fitting. Soft lens showing irregular photokeratogram image.

174 Good fit and PEK image. Good fitting. Soft lens showing regular photokeratogram image.

175 Plus powered soft hydrophilic on eye. Centre thickness of lens = 0.33mm.

N.B. This is a high power plus lens of large optic size.

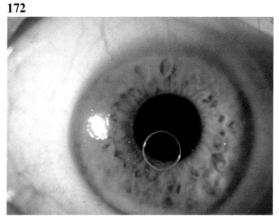

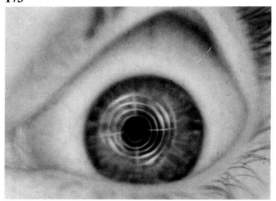

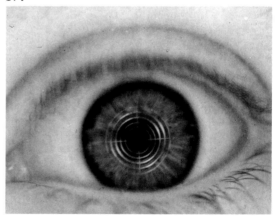

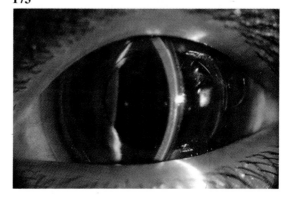

176   Back curves – range of fittings. Back curves, single curves, thin lenses.

Total diameter	Radii					
	7.20	7.60	8.00	8.40	8.80	9.20
12.00	(7.20)	7.60	8.00	8.40	–	–
12.50	7.20	(7.60)	8.00	8.40	–	–
13.00	–	7.60	(8.00)	8.40	8.80	–
13.50	–	7.60	8.00	(8.40)	8.80	–
14.00	–	–	8.00	(8.40)	[8.80]	9.20
14.50	–	–	8.00	8.40	[8.80]	[9.20]
15.00	–	–	8.00	8.40	[8.80]	[9.20]

N.B. This is not designed for keratoconus fittings.

Since soft lens tolerances are big a complete range is rarely required. The lens sizes encircled above are the average fittings in use at this time The radii are equivalent radii and therefore include aspheric back surfaces.

177   Spun moulded lenses (Bausch & Lomb). Essentially fittings are determined by size (sagitta) and mouldability, the other variant thickness. The back curvatures are aspheric. Spun moulded lenses tend to have an oblate elliptical back surface and a front spherical optic. The diagram shows how the liquid polymer mix is spun to form the back curve. High speeds will give steeper back curves.

There is less control by the practitioner with these forms than with lathe cut forms. The same applies to all moulded lenses, i.e. a limitation of fittings. Other examples of moulded lenses are silicone rubber and CAB but the manufacturing process may be injection moulding or pressing of sheet.

177

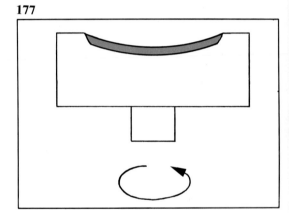

178   Gas permeability and lens thickness. This graph based upon R. Hill (Ohio) data indicates a non-linear relationship of gas transmission properties to thickness. Thus PHEMA (38%) at 0.02mm thick may be as good as a high water content lens (e.g. 60%) of 0.10mm thickness (see bandage lenses).

N.B. Such data are only of experimental value, e.g. thin HEMA 38% water is more likely to dry than a thick polymer of 65% water. The former when dry will rapidly lose its gas permeability properties.

178

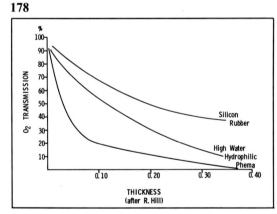

179 Diagrams of lens forms (see Figs. 19–23). Examples of lens form for a low power (−4.00) and high power negative lenses (−25.00). The drawings are in scale.

N.B. Front peripheral lens curves determine lens thickness.

180 Lens forms. A typical back bicurve surface for a low minus −2.00. The thickness is determined by the manufacturing process and material. It could be as thin as 0.04mm at the centre for PHEMA but likely to be 0.12mm in the case of softer materials.

181a Lens forms. Alternative lens designs are shown to control peripheral thickness for high minus lenses. The (a) design uses a front offset negative curve to produce minimal thickness. The lower half (b) compares the conventional positive chamfering with the peripheral front offset.

181b This diagram transfers the lens to the eye shape to show how the thickness is then distributed.

182 Edge form. Soft edge design is mostly determined by the material and method of manufacturing. Very thin edges for some materials is technically difficult.

A shows positive lens edge form. **B** shows negative edge form.

183 Lens forms. For membrane (bandage) lenses to be used as therapeutic lenses the thickness is *optimal* for the manufacturing process and material used. Gas transmission must be able to support corneal metabolism in the closed lid state. HEMA should be avoided even in thin form except for bullous keratopathy.

N.B. These lenses are of large size and low plus powers can be used.

179

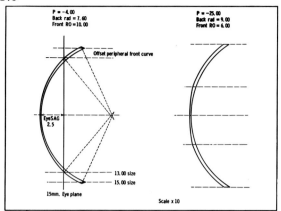

180

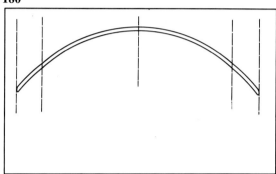

181

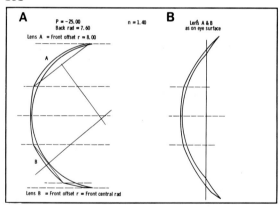

182

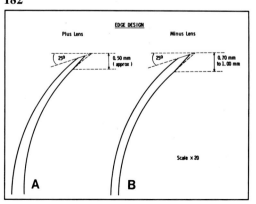

183

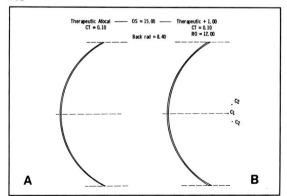

184

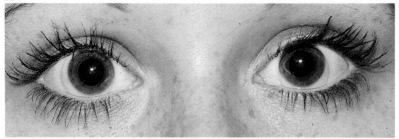

184 Centration problems. Poor centration of soft lenses (low minus).

N.B. Patient is asymptomatic and no tissue response problems and acuity 6/5 each eye.

185

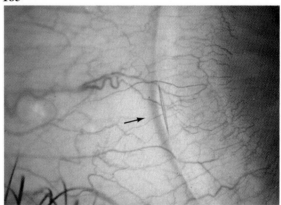

185 Edge fitting problem. Poor edge fitting – too flat.

N.B. Edge is lifting from sclera; also a pinguecula is present.

186

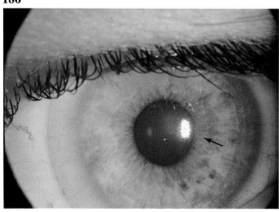

187

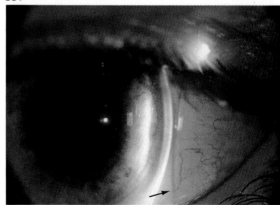

188

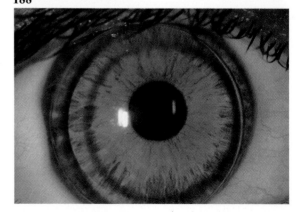

186 & 187 Extended wear gel lens (80% water). Worn by patient for a three year period. Every night he dislodged (Fig. 187) the lens temporally to the sclera.

N.B. Cornea shows epithelial oedema.

188 Silicone rubber lens fittings. Small diameter moulded silicone. Rubber lens (total diameter = 10.80mm) – Danker lens. This shows good centration.

189 Silicone rubber lens fitting. With fluorescein an adequate edge lift and tear fluid exchange is demonstrated on eye movement.

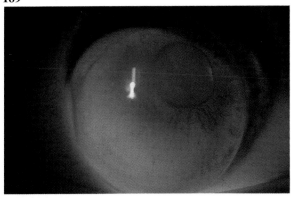

189

190 Silicone rubber lens fitting. With fluorescein this lens shows a tight fit and absence of fluid in peripheral zones. This fit must be avoided for all high powers.

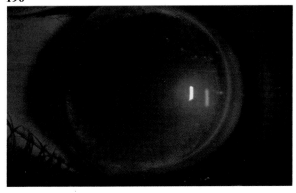

190

191 Toric soft lenses (compare Figs. 117–122).

Types	Front toric or Back toric	powered surfaces
Stabilisers	Toric back surface Conoid back surface Truncations Peripheral toric forms Prism ballast	

One or more combinations of above depending upon position of lower lid to limbus.

In principle maximal stabilisation required for high lower lid positions. Prism ballast not always necessary with truncation.

192 Toric soft lens. Truncation mislocated.

193 Position of truncation or ballast. Truncated lenses will rotate and result in loss of vision.

Types of mislocation: pendular – upon eye movement but 180° in first position; fixed nasal or temporal mislocation; fixed sagging or upriding. Diagram indicates method of recording mislocation.

192

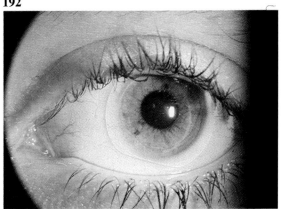

193

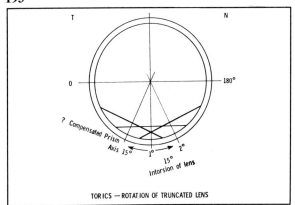

TORICS — ROTATION OF TRUNCATED LENS

193 & 194   Toric soft specification.

K readings:	*K* readings:
Right: 8.20 × 180	Left: 8.30 × 180
7.60	7.50

Spectacle prescription: $\dfrac{-1.00}{-3.00 \times 180}$ Spectacle prescription $\dfrac{-2.50}{-3.50 \times 180}$

Contact lens prescription for front toric truncated lens (PHEMA):

Right: $8.40 : \dfrac{13.00}{14.00}$ | Left: $8.45 : \dfrac{13.00}{14.00}$

power = $-1.00 - 2.50 \times 180$ power = $-2.25 - 3.00 \times 180$

Centre thickness = 0.13mm. Finished lens – lower edge thickness = 0.25mm.

Comment: Right lens acceptable (Fig. 193). Left lens mislocates by 25° (Fig. 194). To be returned for checking, and if correct increased ballast. The power ordered is based upon spectacle over-correction using a trial soft lens of same fitting.

The astigmatic power required for a toric soft lens is almost that of the cornea, but less as the lens rigidity increases (lens thickness and material hardness related).

Note that in high hyperopia the spectacle astigmatic power is less than the corneal and the converse is true for high myopia (due to effectivity).

195   Toric soft fit. Fluorescein stained lens to show degree of mislocation (5°).

N.B. Do not use fluorescein with hydrophilic lenses. This lens is for demonstration only.

196   Toric soft misfit. Note truncation is too high. Therefore lens must be made larger or keeping same size *no* truncation necessary, only prism ballast (1½ △).

197 & 198   Toric lens in version of eye. To show fitting is satisfactory even in extreme versions (Hydron-Europe). Stabilisation of this front toric is obtained by bitruncation without prism ballast. Note that it is often not necessary for prism ballast to be combined with truncation. Distribution of inter-palpebral thickness is the essential factor (e.g. Weicon and Hydrocurve Torics).

197

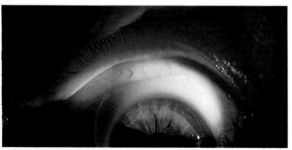

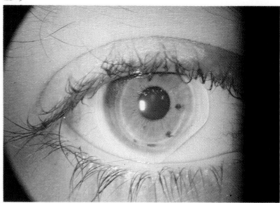

195

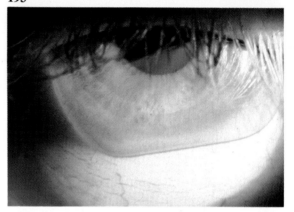

196

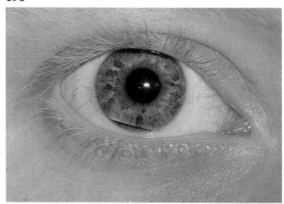

198

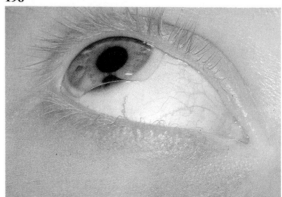

Aphakia and soft lenses

Lens forms (not to scale).
199 Front large optic – 8.50mm diameter, total diameter 14.00mm. Note use of front peripheral negative curves.
200 Front small optic – 7.4mm diameter, total diameter 15.00mm.

201–203 Spun moulded. A 12.50mm spun moulded aphakic correction in PHEMA material.

N.B. Bausch & Lomb fittings now available in 14mm diameters. Side view of Fig. 201 to show good centration and small central front reduced optic (lenticular).

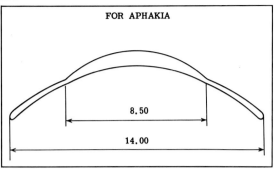

199

FOR APHAKIA

8.50

14.00

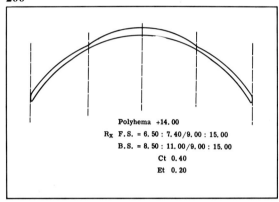

200

Polyhema +14.00
R_X F.S. = 6.50 : 7.40/9.00 : 15.00
B.S. = 8.50 : 11.00/9.00 : 15.00
Ct 0.40
Et 0.20

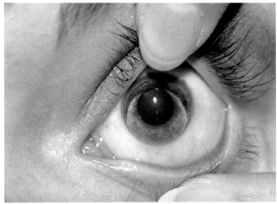

201

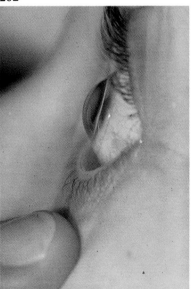

202

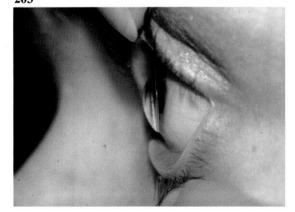

203

204   Lathe cut lens – spherical curves. A 12.50mm lathe cut 75% water content lens worn continuously for four weeks.

204

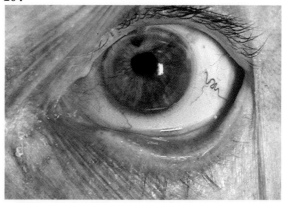

205   Constant wear (cleaning every month and new lenses every six months) for aphakia. Lens fitting 0.60mm flatter than average *K*. Overall lens size 14mm. Peripheral lens thickness 0.15mm. Reduced front optic 8.00mm. Lens water content 75%.

205

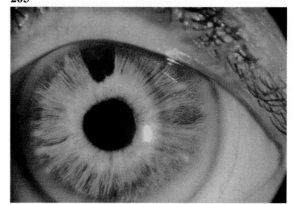

206

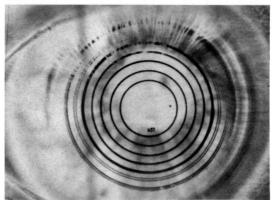

206   PEK of front surface of lens (Fig. 205) to show good image formation and acuity 6/6.

207   Lathe cut lens – spherical curves. A thick 75% water lens worn continuously to show sagging from upper lid pressure.

208   Lathe cut lens – spherical curves. The same lens centres when upper lid is elevated.

208

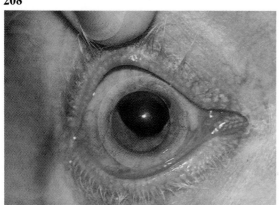

207

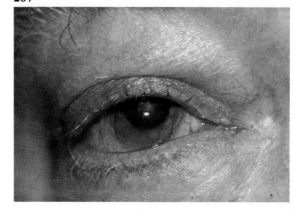

209 Fitting problems. Loose fitting – HEMA lens. Total diameter 13.50mm.

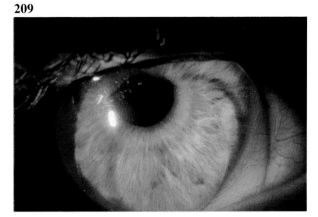

210 Fitting problems. Loose fitting – silicone rubber lens. Total diameter 12.50mm. Temporal slide of lens produces slight optic displacement.

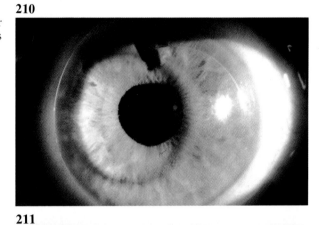

211 Fitting problems. Loose fitting – silicone rubber using fluorescein to assess fitting.

N.B. Optical function may not necessarily be impaired by this fit.

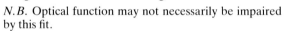

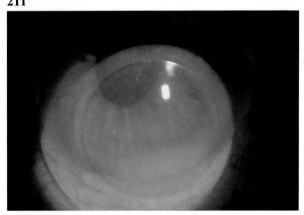

212 Fitting problems. Accurate fitting using silicone rubber lens. Total diameter 12.50mm.

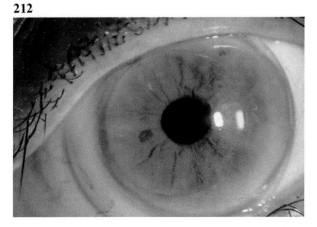

213

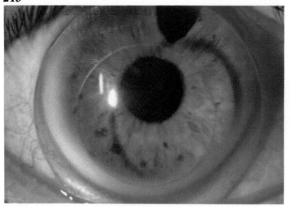

214

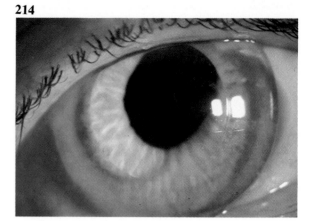

213 & 214 Fitting problems. Acceptable fitting of silicone rubber.

N.B. Silicone lens if too loose causes trauma.

215

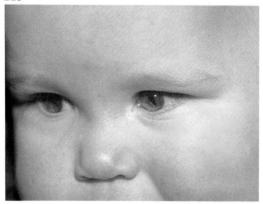

215 Silicone (10.80mm diameter) lenses for aphakic infant (Danker lens).

216

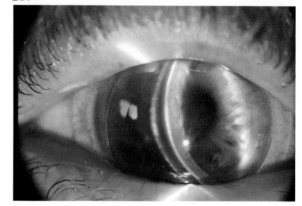

216 Aphakia bullous keratopathy eye fitted with 80% gel (14.50mm diameter) and hard (CAB) lens (7.50mm diameter). The combination was used to provide useful acuity.

Keratoconus and soft lenses

217 Spherical curve, soft lenses. Commercial soft lenses are only of value in early keratoconus and best acuity then with over-correction of a spectacle cylindrical lens. Spherical soft lenses of special design (PHEMA) – fenestrations.

Back curves and sizes: 7.00/13.00
7.40/13.00
7.80/13.50

$$Tc = 0.30$$
$$\overline{Te = 0.16}$$

Front optics must always be reduced.

N.B. Fenestrations to avoid intermediate sealings.

217

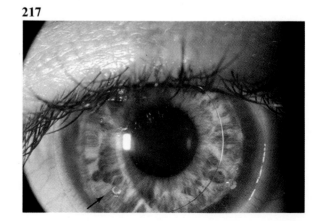

218 & 219 Hard centre soft lenses (combination lens).
(a) Insert type; (b) fused centre of high refractive index;
(c) combination lens. The illustrations show the latter.

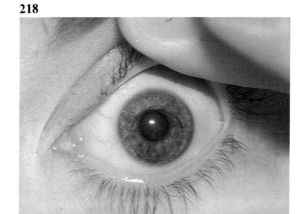

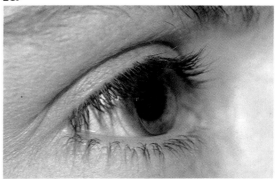

220 Toric soft lens. This will correct residual and
irregular astigmatism Tc =0.25mm.

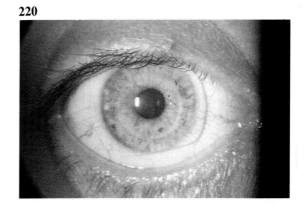

221 Toric truncated gel lens for keratoconus (early)
(Tc =0.25mm).

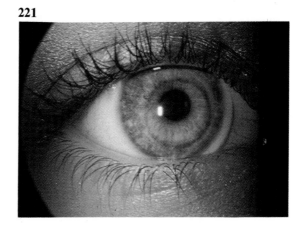

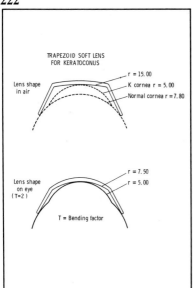

223 Trapezoid back curve design. Trial lenses. Based on BCOR = 12.

1	2	3
12.00 : 8.00	12.00 : 8.50	12.00 : 8.70
8.00 : 14.00	8.00 : 14.00	8.00 : 14.00
9.00 : 15.00	9.00 : 15.00	9.00 : 15.00

power = +2.00 S
Tc   =   0.40 ±0.02
Te   =   0.25
Fenestrations: 4 of 1mm diameter 3mm inset

Material = 38.1 water content.

222 This Trapezoid soft lens illustrates this particular lens form moulding to the eye shape, all soft lenses mould to variable degrees. Thus lens thickness and material determine the relative 'tear lens' effect and therefore power of a soft lens on the eye (bending or wrap factor).

224 Bandage trapezoid. Application of same principle to fit keratoplasty eyes with soft lenses to function as a protective or bandage lens. Based on BCOR = 15.

225 & 226 Trapezoid soft lens (PHEMA). Examples of keratoconus eye wearing a trapezoid fitting.

K readings (Fig. 226): 5.80 → 160 irregular
6.40

Specification of lens fitting (PHEMA):
12.00 : 6.50 two fenestrations
9.00 : 13.50
Tc = 0.35. Power = −4.00.

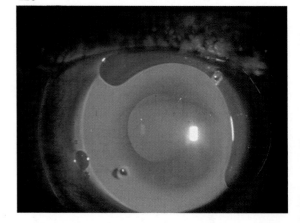

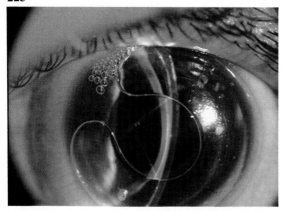

Care of soft lenses

(1) Regularly clean surface with solution and periodic enzyme treatment, (2) store in disinfectant solution, or (3) heat in saline to disinfect.

N.B. Health authorities control the manufacturer by issuing a licence to sell the contact lens and preparations. The practitioner must use the product as indicated by the manufacturer.

227

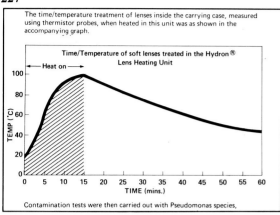

The time/temperature treatment of lenses inside the carrying case, measured using thermistor probes, when heated in this unit was as shown in the accompanying graph.

Time/Temperature of soft lenses treated in the Hydron® Lens Heating Unit

Contamination tests were then carried out with Pseudomonas species,

227 Heat and time period for disinfection. The period of heating in saline can be short periods of high temperatures and pressure (e.g. 130°C for three minutes) or long periods at low temperatures, e.g. 80°C for 40 minutes. The latter is preferred for most materials (courtesy of S&N Research).

228

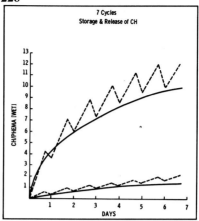

7 Cycles
Storage & Release of CH

228 Chlorhexidine selective lens binding. Cyclic storage of PHEMA in chlorhexidine solution followed by washing in saline does not release all the chlorhexidine since after a few days the chlorhexidine increases in the lens until equilibrium is reached (courtesy of S&N Research). All chemicals used in storage solutions may be irritant to certain patients. Their use is advised with caution, especially in dry eye patients. Chlorhexidine is one example of a chemical disinfectant that binds to the lens material. High water content lenses elute the chemical quickly when worn, but low water content lenses (PHEMA) do so slowly. Thin lenses likewise elute the chlorhexidine over a shorter time. Patient sensitivity to chemicals must be noted.

229

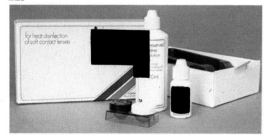

229 Cold solutions and lens case. The lens manufacturer should state preferred method of lens care. It usually involves daily cleaning with a surfactant detergent followed by rinsing and storage; once weekly removal of proteins and lipids by enzyme or solvent preparations. All solutions must be compatible with the lens and case and be relatively non-toxic to the normal eye tissues. Most solutions require a minimum of six hours to disinfect a lens.

230

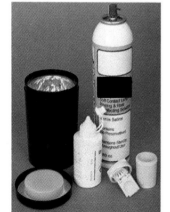

231

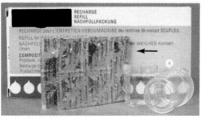

232

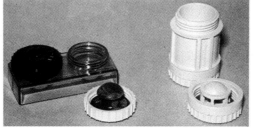

230 Heat-Thermos method. Non-preserved saline is placed in the lens case with the cleaned lenses. The case is sealed with its caps and placed in the Thermos containing just boiled water. The Thermos illustrated is industrial and not easily broken. Electric heaters can also be used. With low temperature heaters just described 40 minutes (or overnight) is required for disinfection.

231 Enzyme tablets are placed in special containers with the lenses and pure water. Agitation and at least 2 hours are required for clean lenses. The enzyme solution must be rinsed off the lens before it is disinfected and worn. The enzyme digests proteinaceous deposits.

232 Gel lens case. Example of badly designed case since the dome does not permit fluid contact with the inside surface of the contact lens.

Scleral fittings

In everyday cosmetic visual practice scleral lenses are not used but for special cases they are still of great value.

> Overall touch – parallel or flush fit.
> Apical minimal touch with limbal clearance and scleral touch.

233 Shapes and sizes. (a) Concentric haptic to optic – for lenses up to 16mm. (b) Nasal displaced optic and oval parameter for all large sizes.

N.B. visual line passes through optic centre which is 0.75mm displaced to geometric centre of optic.

Ventilation is achieved as follows: by loose peripheral fit, or channels in haptic, or fenestrations or slots in limbal zone, and combinations of above methods.

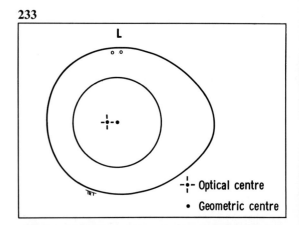

234 Fitting of moulded scleral. Plaster model of eye made from alginate mould of eye. Blue line drawn to indicate parameter.

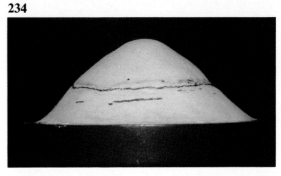

235 Scleral lenses and grafts. Fitting of a moulded scleral – graft eye. For a graft eye, a graduated fluorescein pattern shows that fenestrations or slots must be made where clearance occurs.

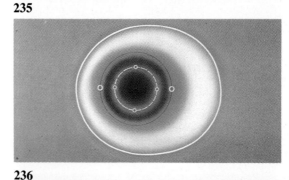

236 Fitting of moulded scleral – marking of the model. Green = back optic position; red = limbal transition; black = parameter of lens.

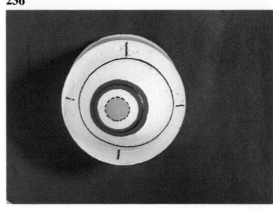

237 Marking of shells. The centre of the shell is marked to guide the placing of the optic back and front curves.

237

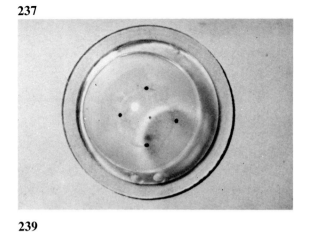

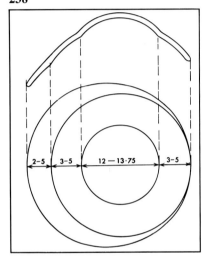

238

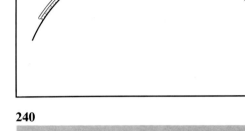

239

238 Lathe cut scleral. By using a solid block of material, multicurve design over several curves can make a geometric scleral lens. Several are necessary to form a fitting set.

239 Ventilated lens – fenestration. Section to show position of fenestrations over zones of clearance.

240 & 241 Ventilated lens – fenestration. With the movement of the eye the lens lifts from the eye because of an edge contact with the globe ligaments. The arrows show a change also of central corneal touch with the lens.

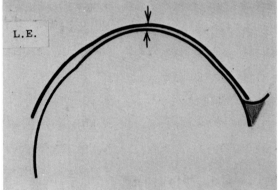

240

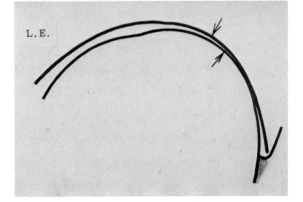

241

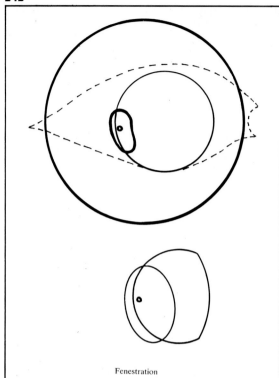

Fenestration

242 Ventilated lens – fenestration. As the lens lifts off the eye and air enters the lens – eye space (lens respiration).

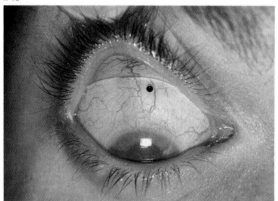

243 Ventilated lens – channel. A channelled lens – this allows supplementary tear lens space fluid to avoid negative pressure.

244 Aphakic scleral lens to show small size of optic.

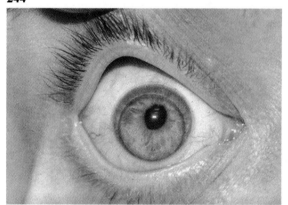

245 Keratoplasty eye scleral lens. Scleral lens fitted to keratoplasty.

N.B. Central touch of graft and lens.

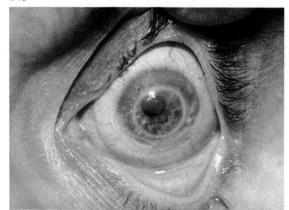

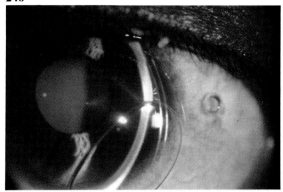

246 Large scleral soft lens. Scleral soft (hydrophilic 38%) lens designed from geometric curves (fenestrated). Horizontal diameter = 25.00mm. Vertical diameter = 22.00mm.

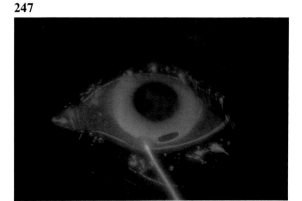

247 Diagnostic scleral lens fitted with silver terminal for electro diagnostic work. Many types of scleral and mini-scleral lenses are used in diagnostic work: 1, Afocal – for acuity testing. 2, Plano front surface – gonioscope and fundus. 3, Spherical front surface (high plus) – Bärkan type gonioscope. 4, Negative front surface (high negative) fundus viewing.

3. Clinical cases

Myopia

248

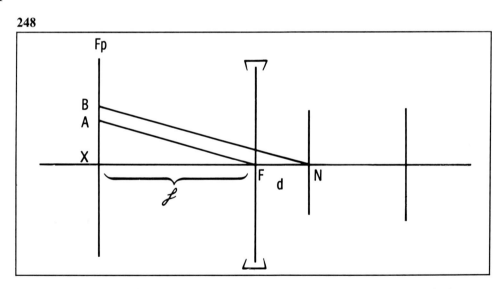

248 Myopia and retinal image size. In axial myopia one can expect a retinal image size increase as compared with spectacles as well as larger field of corrected vision. The increased magnification will therefore give improved acuity for myopia maculopathies.

$$\frac{BX}{AX} = \frac{f + d}{f} = M$$

Example: Spectacle lens = −15.00.
d = 15.00mm.

$$\therefore \ M = \frac{6.81}{6.66} = \times 1.23 \text{ or } 23\% \text{ larger with a contact lens.}$$

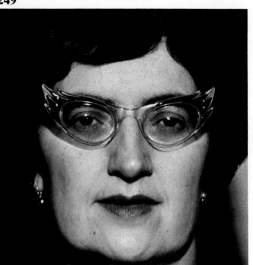

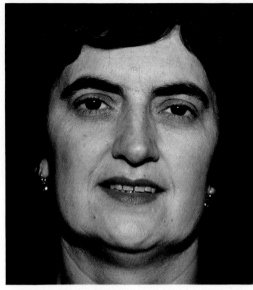

249 Axial degenerative myopia. Degenerative myopia of −19.00 S right and left eyes; woman of 52 years wearing spectacles.

250 Axial degenerative myopia. Same woman wearing hard corneal contact lenses.

Tricurve back surface: 7.80 : 7.80/9.00 : 9.00/12.00 : 9.30.
Tc = 0.08. Te = 0.13.
Reduced optic = 8.00.

251 Pierre Robin syndrome. Small tongue obstructing airway, cleft palate and high myopia (−12.50) – child aged 3½ wearing gel lenses extended wear.

251

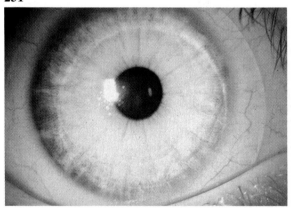

252 Congenital myopia. A 4-year-old child fitted with daily wear HEMA 38% hydrophilic lenses.

8.50/13.00 – 9.00.
Tc = 0.10. Te = 0.12.
Front optic = 8.50.

252

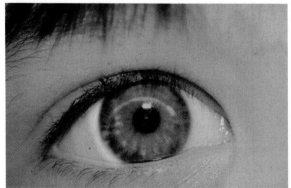

Regular and irregular astigmatism

253 Photokeratograph showing regular corneal image outline of normal myopic (simple myopia) fitted with corneal hard contact lens.

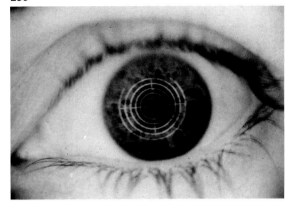

254 Keratoplasty. Regular astigmatism of a keratoplasty fitted with hard corneal lens.

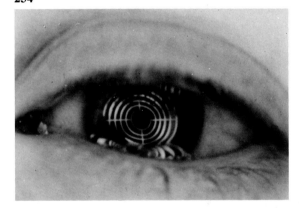

255 Keratoplasty. Irregular astigmatism of keratoplasty – intolerant to hard lens and fitted with Hema (38%) soft lens daily wear.

> Acuity with hard lens = 6/6.
> Acuity with soft lens = 6/12.
> Centre thickness of soft lens specially designed to give rigidity ($Tc = 0.20$ $Te = 0.16$).
> Front optic reduced to 10mm.
> Power = −2.00. Total diameter = 13.50mm.

256 Myopic astigmatism. A Right eye photokeratogram shows regular astigmatism (myopic astigmatism −2.00 S −2.00 cyl. axis 180°).

  B Left eye. Corneal scarring from ulceration – note irregular astigmatism. Eye not fitted.

  Acuity = 6/18 with −1.75 S; with trial contact lens = 6/9.

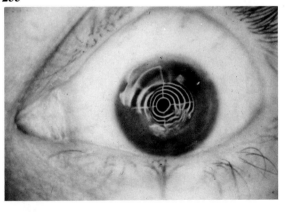

256a

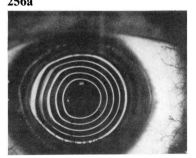

256b

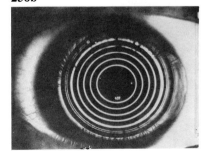

257 Keratoconus. Irregular astigmatism of early keratoconus fitted with hard corneal gas permeable contact lens.

> Prescription: 7.30 : 6.50 peripheral offset
> with axial edge lift 0.15
>
> Total diameter = 9.00.
> $Tc = 0.12$. $Te = 0.18$.
> Power = −5.00.

N.B. Back curve is pseudo-conoidal contour.

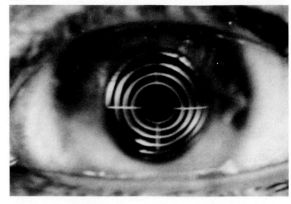

258 Lamellar keratoplasty. 10mm lamellar graft for treatment of herpetic keratitis fitted with hard scleral because of associated dry eye. Acuity with contact lens = 6/12. Acuity with spectacles = 6/36. Unaided acuity = 4/60.

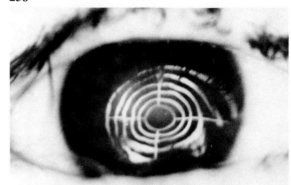

258

259 Graft elevation. Inferior graft elevation with distortion fitted with hard scleral contact lens. Acuity with best spectacles = 6/60. Acuity with contact lens = 6/9.

260 Keratoconus keratoplasty. Penetrating keratoplasty for keratoconus. Acuity unaided = 6/6.
Compare with photokeratograph of Fig. 255.

261 Marginal ulceration (possibly Moorens type). Soft lens and steroids during active phase. But scleral hard to give acuity five years after onset of condition.

259

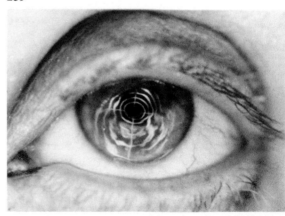

261

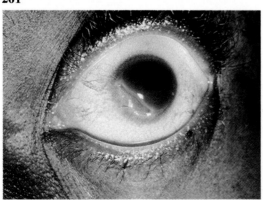

260

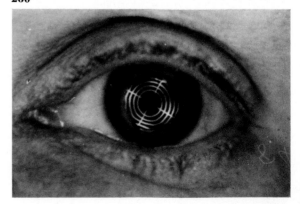

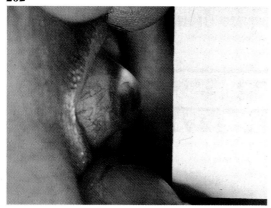

262 A keratoglobus eye. Note sphericity over total diameter.

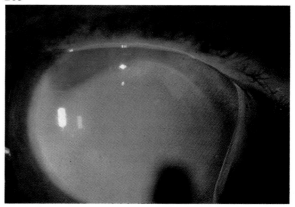

263 A keratoglobus eye. The eye is fitted with a scleral lens which is the only type to use in this condition.

Aphakia

264 Optics of aphakia. Ametropia, eye length and keratometry.

$$\text{Ametropia} = \text{Ax} - K = \frac{1.333 \times 10^3}{L} - K$$

$$K = \frac{0.37 \times 10^3}{r}$$

Ax = axial power of eye

L = axial length of eye

K = keratometric power in dioptres

r = radius of curvature of corneal optic zone

When Ax = K = pseudo-emetropic state.
This occurs when the eye has high degrees of axial myopia (approximately −18.00).

265 Choice of contact lens.

Hard corneal:
good acuity;
corrects astigmatism;
possibility of near vision.

Hard scleral:
for abnormal corneal contours and lid anomalies.

Soft:
best acuity if residual astigmatism corrected by spectacles;
good tolerance – extended wear a possibility.

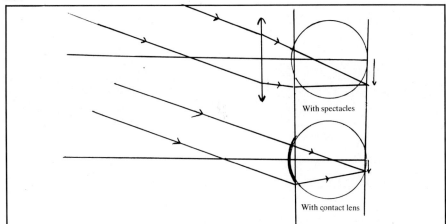

266 Image size. The size of the image produced by a spectacle lens is 20–30% for the emetropic aphakic eye. The contact lens reduces this to 2–10%. The pseudo-lens implant can produce +2% to −5%.

267 **Simulated image size differences.** A street scene is visualised with a camera corrected by an aphakic spectacle correction and then with an equivalent contact lens correction. The photograph on the right is with the spectacle correction and that on the left with the contact lens. *Contact Lens Practice* (See M. Ruben (1975) Bailliere Tyndall, London).

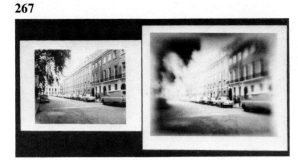

268 **Principal optical factors in development.** Whilst the corneal curvatures in the axial zone change very little with growth from birth to adult, the eye size and position of the crystalline lens changes considerably, especially in the first three years of life.

269 **Eye size in infancy.** Aphakic eye length at birth and at age four.

270 **Ametropia in irfancy.** Aphakic ametropia is much greater than in the adult. The graph gives approximate powers.

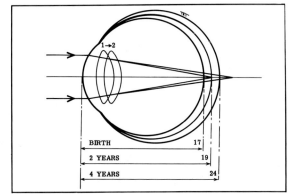

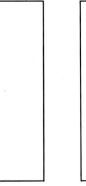

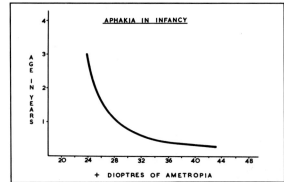

271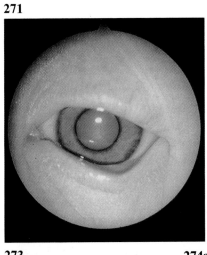

272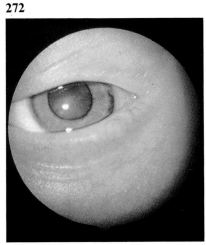

271 & 272 Total cataract at birth. A baby born with total cataract of both eyes.

273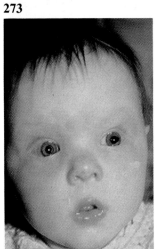

274a Right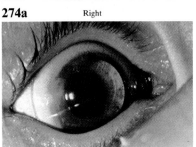

274b Left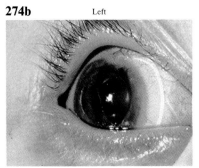

273, 274a & 274b Wearing contact lenses. After removal of the cataracts both eyes are fitted with hydrophilic (75% H$_2$O) soft lenses for continuous wear. Note that the lenses are larger than the corneal diameter (13.50mm). (Figs. 271–274 a patient of D. Taylor FRCS.)

275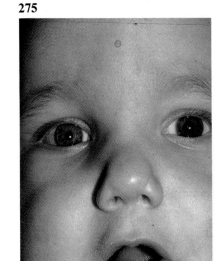

276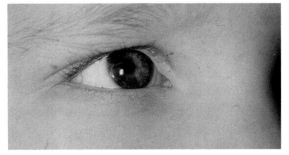

275 & 276 Infant aphakic wearing contact lens. Another example of bilateral aphakia in infancy wearing hydrophilic soft lenses (75% water content).

277 Adult aphakic with spectacles. Reduced optic spectacle correction to show limitations of corrected vision.

278 Adult aphakic with contact lenses. Same patient corrected by hard corneal lenses.

Back surfaces: 7.50 : 7.00/9.00 : 8.70/12.00 : 9.20. Power = +14.00. Front optic diameter = 8.70.

N.B. Front optic diameter is larger than back central optic – this gives better near vision.

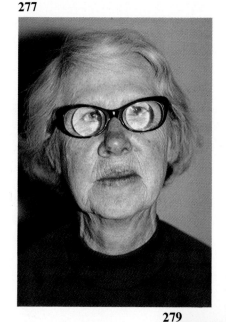

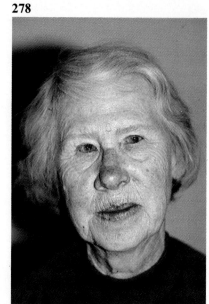

279 Adult aphakic and extended wear. A continuous wear gel (75% water) lens to correct woman aged 65.

Prescription: back curve: 8.70 : 14.00. Power = +18.00. $Tc = 0.54$. Reduced optic = 8.00. $Te = 0.18$.

This is a *loose* fit gel lens. Essential for extended wear with this material.

279
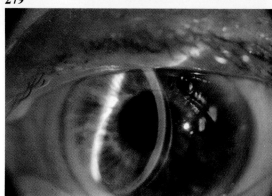

280
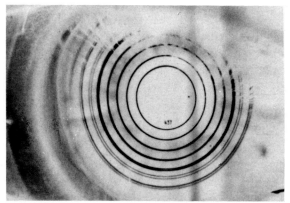

280 Photokeratograph of lens (gel). Photokeratograph of the above lens surface when on the eye. Regular circles with little astigmatism.

281
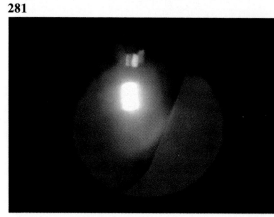

281 Subluxed lens (Marfan's Syndrome) (arachnodactyly). The aphakic portion is corrected by a contact lens.

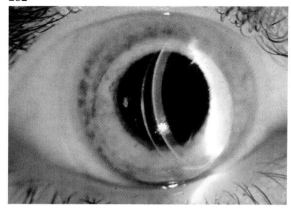

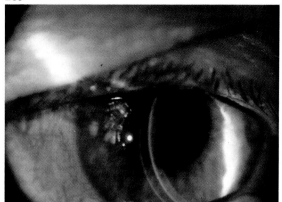

282 High hypermetropia in a child (hereditary). Gel (38% water) daily wear.

Prescription: 8.60 : 9.00/9.00 : 13.00. Power = +18.00. Reduced front optic = 8.50mm. *T*c = 0.60. *T*e = 0.16.

N.B. 1. Centre thickness greater than corneal thickness – anoxia of the cornea is a possibility.
N.B. 2. The back curve is of bicurve design because of unusual thickness of the lens. The bicurve design will assist flexibility.

283 Hypermetropic adult. Female aged 50 wearing gel (45%) lens +2.50 power. Average keratometry = 7.25.

Prescription: back curve = 8.20/12.50. *T*c = 0.50. Single curve lenses, no front reduced optic.

284 Keratoconus (see Chapter 2 – fitting procedures). Keratoconus is an important condition in contact lens practice. Good acuity is possible except in severe degrees. Hard lenses give best acuity. In principle the size of the lens fitted increases as the curvature steepens.

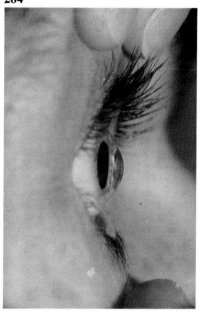

Albinism

285 Examples of occlusion. Occlusion lens with clear pupil area of sizes 9–13mm. Used in albinism, congenital and secondary total and partial aniridia, for cosmetic and prosthetics (see Chapter 6).

286 Examples of occlusion. Haptic lens occluded except for pupillary aperture. This form also possible in scleral size especially as a prosthetic lens (see Chapter 6).

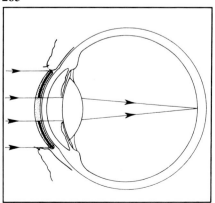

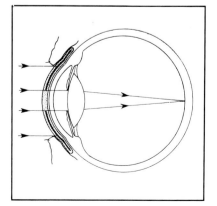

287

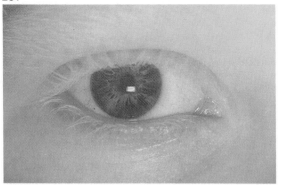

287 An albino eye. Note the chorio-retinal reflected light in iris and pupil.

288

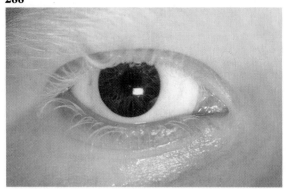

288 An albino eye. The same eye fitted with an occlusive scleral lens, i.e. back surface of lens is black and front white – pupil is clear.

N.B. Very difficult to tolerate. Alternative lenses are colour print soft and homogeneous tinted soft.

Anirida

289

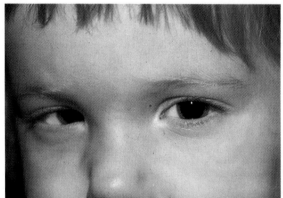

289–291 Congenital aniridia. Brown iris Weicon lenses successfully worn bilaterally.

290

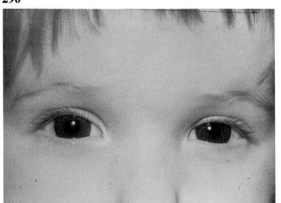

291

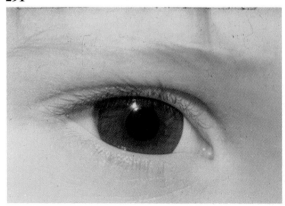

Acne rosacea keratitis

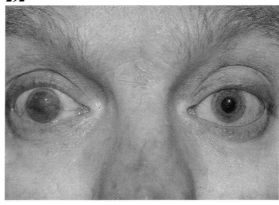

292 & 293   Scleral hard lens. Fitted to give best acuity. Cornea shows scarring and vascularisation. Soft lens proved of no visual value.

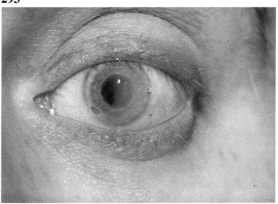

Corneal dystrophy

294   Corneal dystrophy. A non-inflammatory marginal stromal lysis between Bowman's membrane and limbus. Results in irregular central astigmatism with flat corneal curves. Diagnosis was Terrien's Dystrophy.

N.B. Difficult to fit with small hard lenses. Fitted with hard scleral or toric soft lenses.

295 & 296   Macular corneal dystrophy.
   In early stages visual improvement with various types of lens possible. In later phase keratoplasty is done but recurrence of metabolic dysfunction is often seen in the keratoplasty. Grafted eye. Fig. 296 fitted with hard corneal.

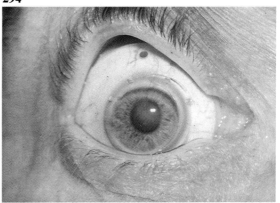

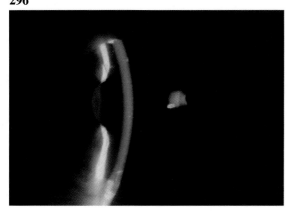

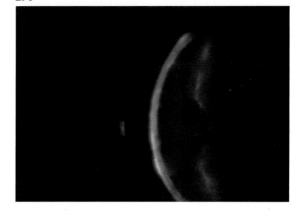

Trachoma with dry eye

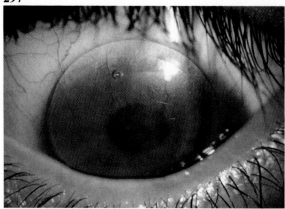

297 Trachoma pannus and keratitis with dry eye problems. Trachoma is associated with lid anomalies, secretion and tear deficiency. Soft hydrophilic lenses do not succeed in advanced cases; this patient succeeded with better vision with silicone rubber lenses (size 10.80mm).

Progressive myopathy

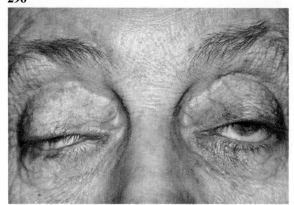

298 & 299 Progressive myopathy of ocular muscles. Female aged 75 wearing ptosis props to obtain vision.

300 Ptosis. Ptosis lid occlusive lens with painted iris to avoid insuperable diplopia.

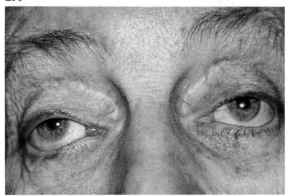

Sub-normal vision aid

301 The eye can be fitted with a high negative powered lens and the vision corrected by a suitable positive powered spectacle lens.

$$\text{Magnification} = \frac{1}{1 - dF}$$

where d = spectacle distance and F = power of spectacle lens.

Therefore the bridge fitting of the spectacles must bring forward the spectacles as much as possible.

Suggest BVD = 20–25mm. Suggest contact lens produce ocular ametropia of 10–15 hyperopia.

301

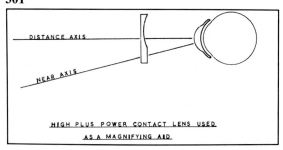

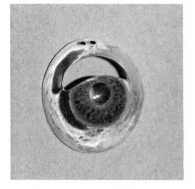

Binocular vision indications

1. To achieve and maintain binocular single vision in: anisemetropia and aniseikonia, latent strabismus, and strabismus.

2. To occlude the eye: by optical (partial and selective), or depression of light stimulus.

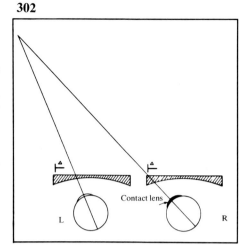

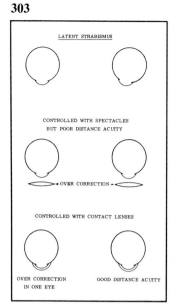

302 **Combined contact and spectacle lenses** – principle of contact lens partial correction of highly ametropic eye with balancing spectacles. Unilateral aphakia treated with contact lens and spectacles to produce *relative* prismatic effects and reduction of aniseikonia. The left phakic eye is myopic and cannot tolerate a contact lens.

303 **Heterophoria and contact lens over-correction.** Latent strabismus corrected by use of over-correction contact lenses in less dominant eye.

304 **Alternating convergent strabismus (and hyperopia).** Tropia with spectacles = +12°. Tropia without spectacles = +22°. Tropia with contact lenses using *one* eye with distance correction and the other eye +1.50 S over-correction = 7°.

Soft or hard corneal can be used providing centration is good and tolerance satisfactory.

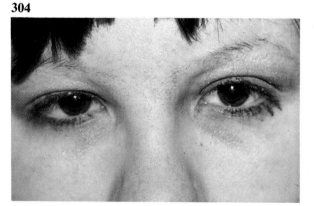

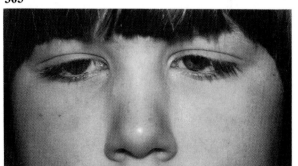

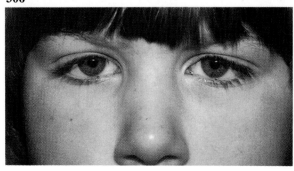

305 & 306 **Alternating convergent strabismus.** Child aged 8 years, left convergent strabismus – patient without contact lenses and accommodating. +5.00 hyperopia each eye. Below same patient as Fig. 305 with soft daily wear contact lenses and accommodating.

307

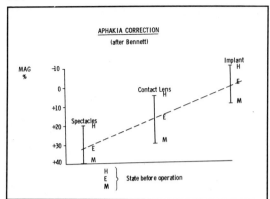

308

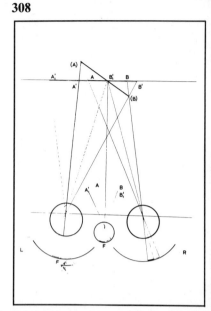

307 Unilateral aphakia. To show the difference in image size between an aphakic and other eye supposing the pre-aphakic state to be known.

308 Aniseikonia. The different retinal sizes result in fusion only if the projected image departs from the front-parallel plane. Thus the new plane appears tilted with reference to the true plane.

309–311 Measurement of aniseikonia. Ruben's synoptophore slides (based upon Ames-Ogle Ikeinometer). The doubling of the vertical line on one side only determines the presence of aniseikonia and this can subsequently be measured. Fig. 309 shows the tilted front-parallel plane with fusion.

309

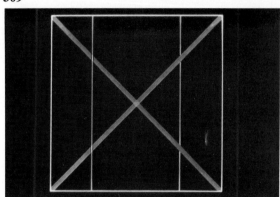

310

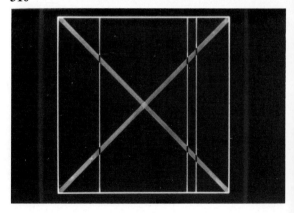

311

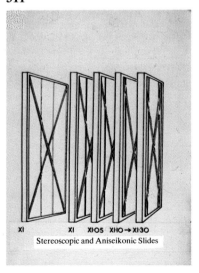

312 Traumatic unilateral aphakia. Unilateral aphakia of traumatic aetiology corrected by adhesive corneal lens. (Technique now obsolete.)

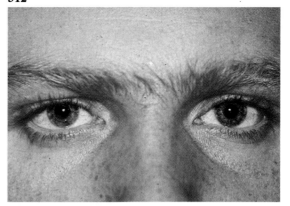

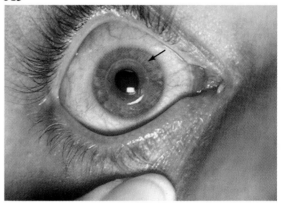

313 Traumatic unilateral aphakia. The corneal adhesive lens *in situ*. Orthoptic examination demonstrated that conventional contact lens did not give binocular single vision but adhesive lens did.

Conclusion. A contact lens to produce good binocular single vision in anisometropia must maintain good centration.

314 Intra-ocular lens implant in young woman (aged 26) producing good binocular single vision after traumatic cataract and aphakia. Patient had failed to wear contact lenses. Implant was secondary insertion. Twelve years after insertion the nylon loops degenerated and broke with tilting of the implant.

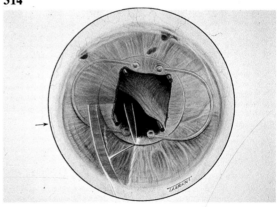

314 Optical occlusion using contact lenses producing selective myopic state. Therefore distance vision in good eye is occluded, but not for using negative power contact lenses hyperopia for both distance and near vision is produced with optical central occlusion near.

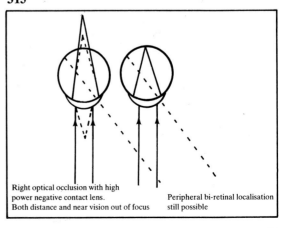

Right optical occlusion with high power negative contact lens. Both distance and near vision out of focus

Peripheral bi-retinal localisation still possible

315 Optical occlusion using negative powered lens produces a hyperopic state and acute foveal image stimulus not possible.

316

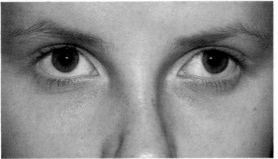

317

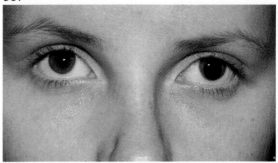

316 & 317 Paralytic strabismus. A patient with divergent strabismus and diplopia of neurological aetiology. Same patient wearing an occlusive contact lens of hydrophilic material (left eye).

318

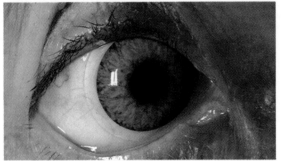

318 Coloured occlusive lens. Using a coloured soft gel to have also a cosmetic effect.

319

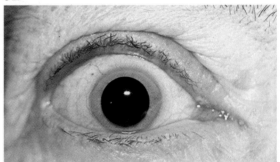

319 Occlusive pupil contact lens. Another example of a pupil occlusive lenses (soft gel).

Dry eyes and exposure problems

320, 321 & 322 Familial dysautonomia (Riley–Day syndrome). Congenital inherited anomaly of autonomic system with loss of tears and diminished sensation. Six years of hydrophilic soft lens wear using 75% water gel.

321 Same case a few months later.

320

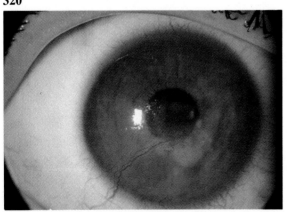

321

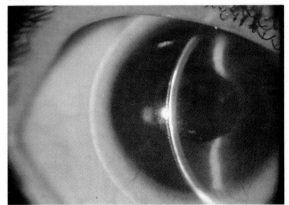

322 Familial dysautonomia. Same case six years later.

N.B. Vascularisation and scarring of cornea compensated. Ancillary eye treatment with paraffin drops and paraffin eye ointment (Lacrilube). Non-wetting of lens surface due to oily drops.

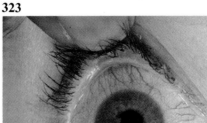

323 & 324 Vth cranial nerve lesion. In both instances the eye is completely anaesthetic owing to Vth cranial nerve lesion (intra-cranial). Note corneal scarring and vascularisation. Soft lenses used during day and lids closed by Blenderm tape at night. Problems emanate from the dry eye and abnormal tear reflexes.

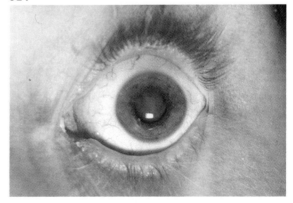

325 & 326 Pityriasis rubra. Patient has recurrent corneal ulceration.

326 Same patient with eye closed showing exposure problem. Patient treated with hard scleral; soft lenses dried and caused intolerance.

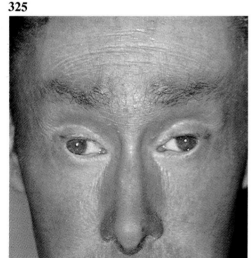

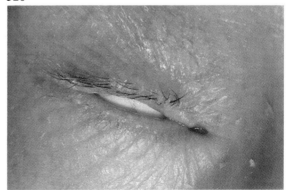

327 Lid ectropia and exposure keratitis. Ectropia and exposure keratitis with corneal vascularisation and lipid infiltration. Only scleral hard of value or plastic surgery (refused by patient).

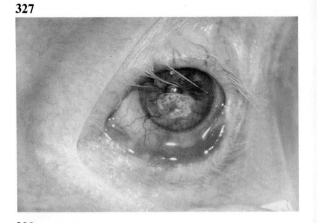
327

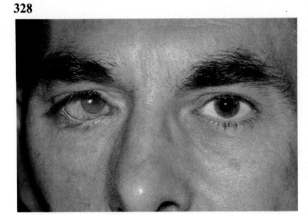
328

328, 329 & 330 VIIth cranial nerve lesion. Facial paralysis right side and left amblyopic eye. Right scleral lens worn constantly, removed approximately every eight hours.

N.B. Soft hydrophilic lens contra-indicated because of rapid drying.

329 Eyes closed.

N.B. Bell's reflex seen in right eye.

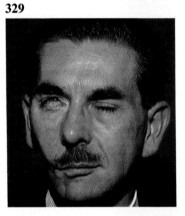
329

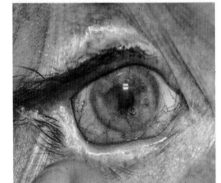
330

330 Ten years later.

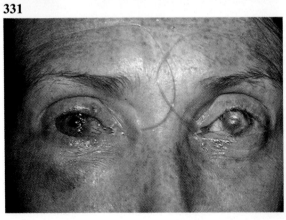
331

331 Stevens–Johnson syndrome (erythema multiforme). Patient with bilateral capillary perfusion of both eyes with Ringer's solution.

332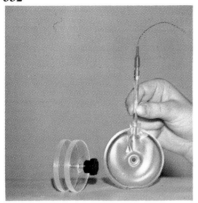

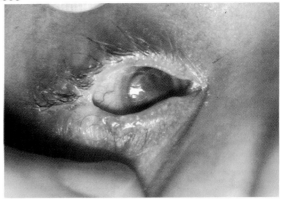

332 Perfusion tank with pressure controlled by thumb screw and plastic plates.

333 Stevens–Johnson syndrome. Right eye of a patient most severely affected by Stevens–Johnson syndrome treated by tarsorraphy and artificial tears.

334 Stevens–Johnson syndrome. Less serious than above patient some two years after attack fitted with high water content bandage lens. Note trichiasis of upper lid.

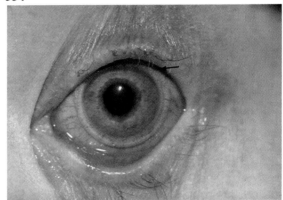

335 Ocular pemphigoid (benign mucous membrane atrophy). Hard lens (PMMA – size 13.00mm).
   Back curves: $8.40 : 8.40/9.00 : 13.00$. $Tc = 0.10$. Power – plano. $Te = 0.10$.
   Lens wear purpose was to retain fluid behind lens and give some subjective improvement in vision. 'Liqui' tear drops inserted every ten minutes to prevent keratinisation of cornea.

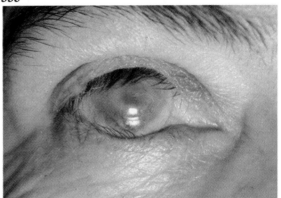

336 Ocular pemphigoid (benign mucous membrane atrophy). Patient was fitted with moulded scleral. Soft hydrophilic are contra-indicated, and silicone rubber became surface spoiled.

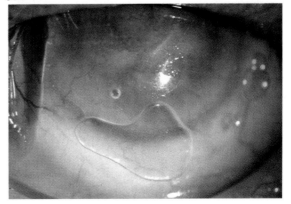

337 **Symblepharon** divided in ocular pemphigoid and ring (scleral) of PMMA inserted.

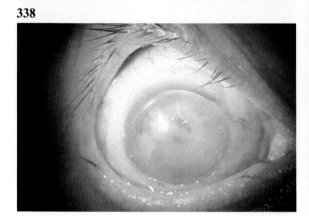

338 & 339 **Stevens–Johnson dry eye syndrome (erythema multiforme).** The eye fitted with clear pupil prosthetic shell to maintain fornices.

N.B. Trichiasis.

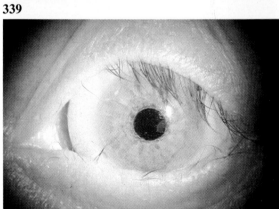

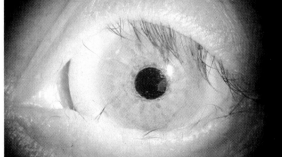

340 **Intractable lid entropion and trichiasis.** Corneal scarring from lid entropion (cicatricial) and trichiasis. Alleviated by hydrophilic soft lens. Surgical procedures to correct trichiasis should be considered but can cause exposure problems.

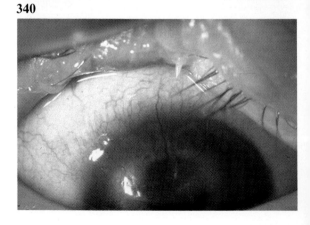

341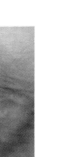

342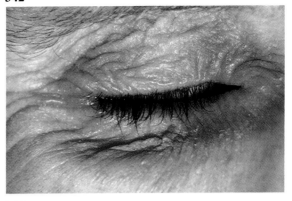

341 & 342 Facial hemiatrophy. Facial atrophy and exposure keratitis. Ring (scleral) to form pseudo-lid margin and maintain tear meniscus. Showing the eye open and closed.

343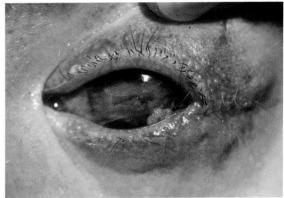

343 & 344 Buphthalmos. Buphthalmos and endothelial degeneration with secondary chronic corneal oedema and infective keratitis (only eye).

Same eye three years later wearing bandage hydrophilic soft lens.

Prescription of back curve:
8.90 : 8.00
10.00 : 13.00
11.00 : 15.00

Tc = 0.12. Te = 0.13. Power = −1.00. Material 60% water content.

344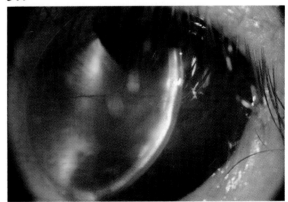

345 Buphthalmos (only eye). Fitted with hard moulded scleral lens (acuity 6/60). Soft lens tried but abandoned because of poor acuity.

346 Recurrent corneal erosion. Large recurrent erosion of cornea treated by keratectomy and large thin gel bandage lens.

346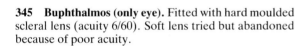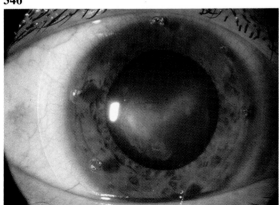

345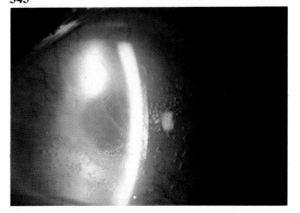

347 Graft elevation and pain with blepharospasm. The eye was treated with gel bandage lens. Note the stromal lysis in the host cornea.

347

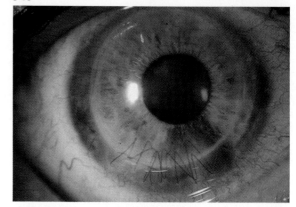

348 Graft elevation (below). This was treated by criss-cross suturing and gel bandage lens.

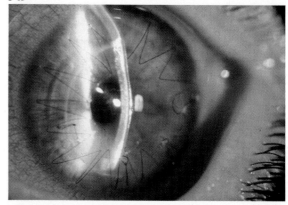

349 Keratoplasty. Graft covered by trapezoid and bandage lens at end of operation and worn for several weeks post-operatively (see Trapezoid Soft Lenses, page 64).

Prescription of back curve:
15.00 : 8.00
9.00 : 15.00

Tc = 0.10. Te = 0.10. Power – plano. 85% (Sauflon) water content.

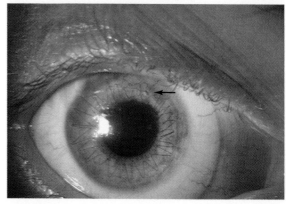

350 Keratoplasty. Penetrating graft with 10.00's Perlon sutures which became loose one month after operation. Bandage gel lens was worn for two weeks until sutures were removed.

Prescription of lens:
76% water gel
back curve: 8.80 : 9.00
10.00 : 13.00
12.00 : 16.00
Tc = 0.12. Te = 0.15.

Note extra large size of lens.

Bullous keratopathy

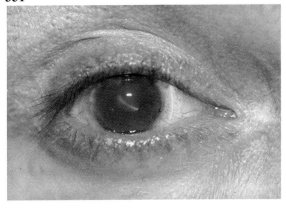

351 Bullous keratopathy. Right anterior chamber pseudo-lens implant (aphakic eye). Endothelial dysfunction and chronic corneal oedema with bullae of epithelium. Treated with soft bandage lens.

352 Left eye of the same patient with anterior chamber implant and minimal endothelial dysfunction.

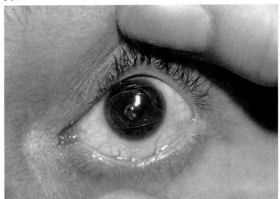

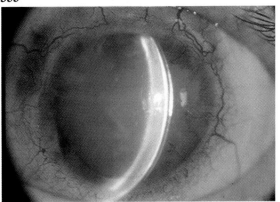

353 Bullous keratopathy after cataract extraction. Treated with soft bandage lens.

354 Combination hard and soft. Soft with hard lens to give better acuity for bullous keratopathy. The hard lens can be of gas permeable material.

355 & 356 Adhesive hard lens (obsolete). A precursor of the extended wear soft lens, before operation. (*See* Fig. 480 for diagram of method.)

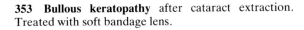

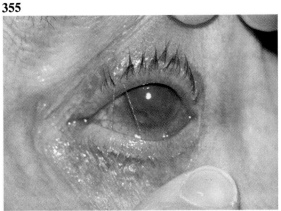

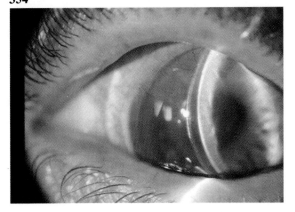

356 Adhesive hard lens (obsolete). This treatment removed the dead epithelium and replaced it with a hard corneal lens made adherent at the edge with cyanoacrylate glues.

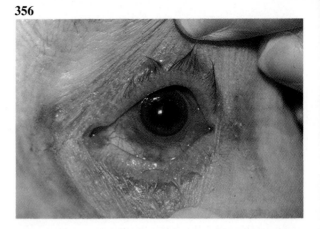

357 New vessels in bullous keratopathy. Bullous keratopathy showing complication of new vessel formation. After six months of continuous wear the lens is removed. If no further pain stop wear. If pain persists continue wear. If vision required penetrating graft has 50% success rate over a three year post-operation period.

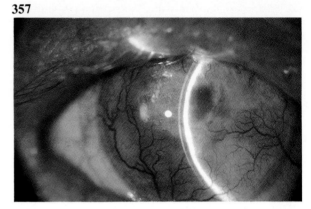

358 & 359 Mesodermal dysplasia and endothelial dysfunction. Note folds in endothelium of this congenital condition, and chronic corneal oedema. The patient was a gel lens wearer for temporary period but most successful with scleral hard lens (359).

N.B. Hard lens will give better visual result than soft lens.

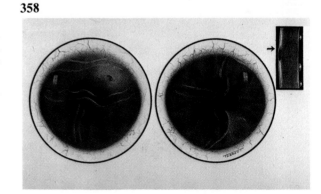

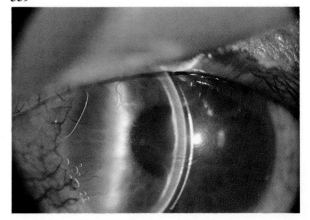

Soft lens glaucoma treatment (drug dispenser soft lens)

360

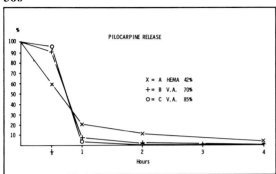

360 Rates of drug release of different contact lens materials, (Pilocarpine).

361

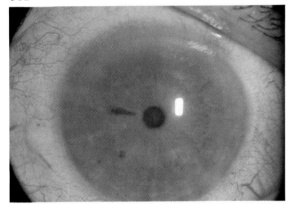

361 Gel lens dispenser on eye. Glaucomatous eye with gel soaked pilocarpine lens showing good miosis ten hours after insertion.

Anterior chamber reformation

362

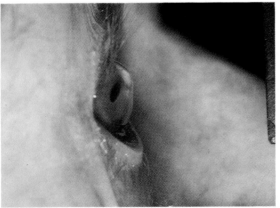

363

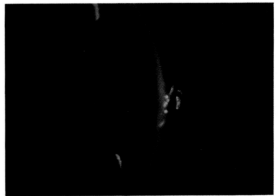

362 Perforating megalocornea. Patient fitted with large gel bandage lens to restore anterior chamber.

363 & 364 Perforating corneal wounds. Two examples of puncture wounds of cornea reformed anterior chambers only after bandage lens was used.

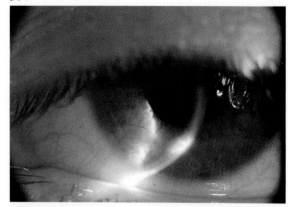
364

365 & 366 Perforating cornea. Front and slit-lamp view of corneal perforation treated with bandage gel lens.

365

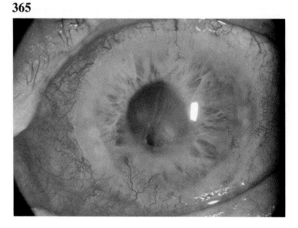

366

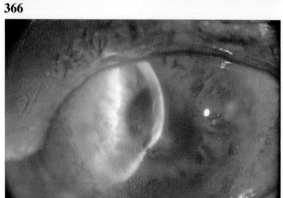

Herpes simplex and anti-viral dispenser

367 & 368 Herpes simplex (recurrent episodes). Same eye treated with anti-viral chemotherapy (one tenth normal drop concentration) dispensed from bandage gel lens.

Note lens fenestrations to allow local therapy.

367

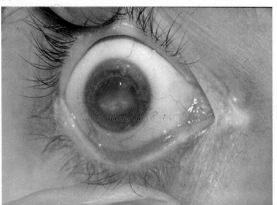

368

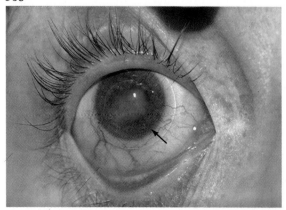

369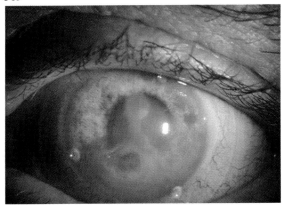

370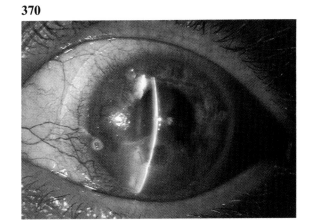

369 & 370 Herpes simplex (recurrent episodes). Front and slit-beam views of cornea of metaherpetic corneal ulceration and corneal perforation treated with soft bandage lens prior to lamellar graft operation.

The bandage lens

371 Bandage lens materials and permeability to 0₂ and hardness.

		Thickness	O_2*	Hardness
Sauflon	85% Polyvinyl acrylate	0.12	68	1.50
Hoya	75% Polyvinyl acrylate	0.10	55	2.00
Bausch & Lomb	38% HEMA	0.04	30	2.50

*DK Units.
Hardness is relative to PMMA at 100.

372 Lens form for a therapeutic bandage gel lens. Centre thickness depends upon material rigidity – thus HEMA can be 0.04mm thick, but Sauflon, Duragel, Perma, material 0.10mm or more (all high water content materials). See Fig. 373 for thickness of lens and form.

Specifications

Material: Duragel 75%
$Tc = 0.12$
Back curve $= 8.50$
Total diameter $= 15.00$
Power $= +0.75$ (± 0.25)

373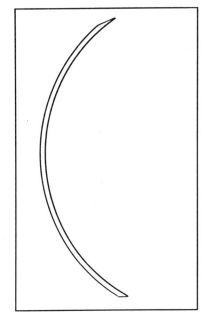

Burns of eye

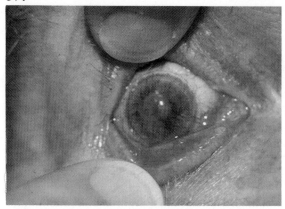

374 Mustard gas keratitis. Elderly patient with cornea now undergoing secondary degeneration.

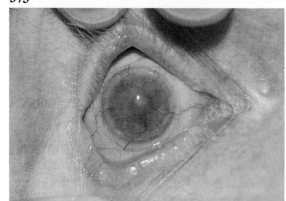

375 Mustard gas keratitis. Improvement of right eye after two weeks of soft gel lens wear.

376, 377 & 378 Chemical burns – caustic soda type. Treated by graft and bandage lens. Resulted in a quiet, comfortable eye.

377 One year after treatment.

378 Two and a half years after treatment.

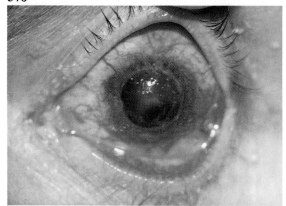

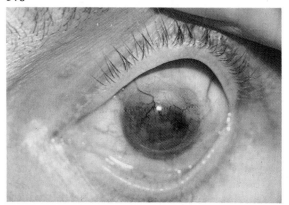

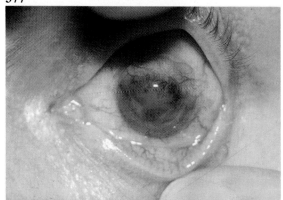

379

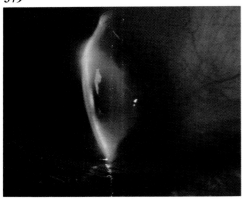

379 Ammonia burn. Severe ammonia burn with melting cornea. Bandage lens used to alleviate pain – eye eventually enucleated.

380

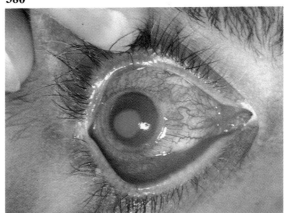

380 Ammonia burn. Treated with gel lens and irrigation.

Conformer rings and synechia

381

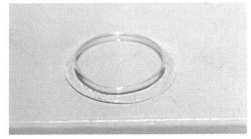

382

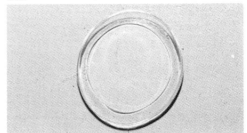

381 & 382 Use of conformer rings to maintain fornices. Rings cut from a scleral shell of PMMA material – soft materials can also be used.

383

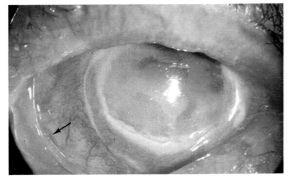

383 Conformer rings *in situ*. Lime burn – several weeks after accident with scleral ring in position.

384

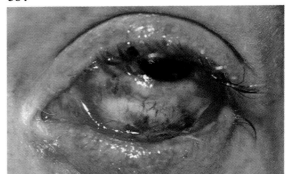

384 Conformer rings *in situ*. A ring in position and showing scleral necrosis.

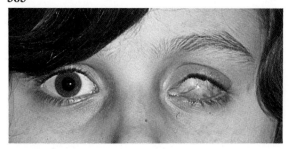

385

385 Conformer rings *in situ*. Lime burn with symblepharon.

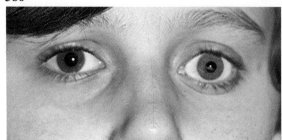

386

386 Cosmetic shell as fornix conformer. Cosmetic shell *in situ* after division of symblepharon.

387 Further examples of chemical burns. Chemical burn – lime.

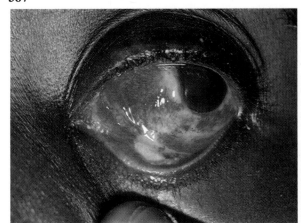

387

388 & 389 Chemical burns treated with conforming rings.

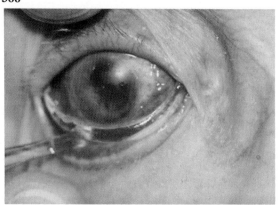

388

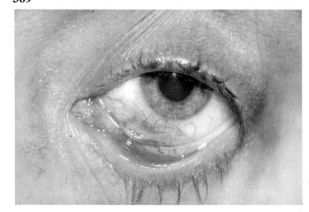

389

390 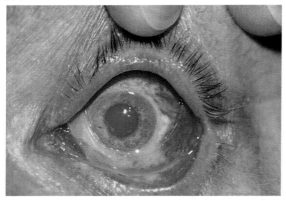 **391**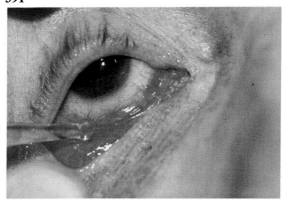

390 & 391 Chemical burns treated with conforming rings – further examples.

392 – 395 Molten brass burn treated with ring.

392 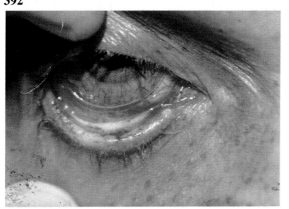 **393**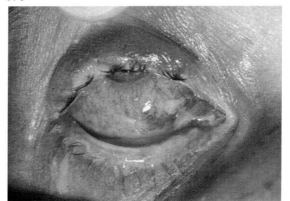

394 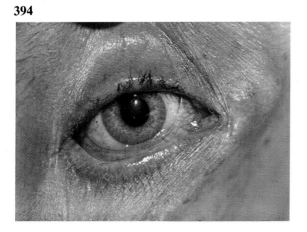 **395**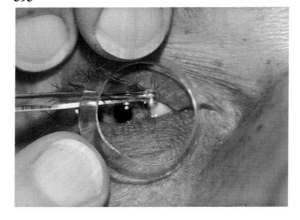

396 Molten brass burn treated with ring. The patient retained a conformer ring for three months and had local treatment with steroids and antibiotics. Note plaque formation lower lid.

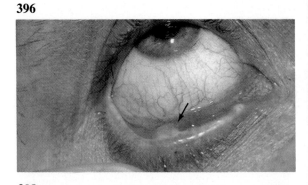

396

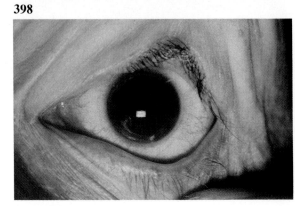

397

398

397 & 398 Burns of face and lid grafts. The end result was corneal distortion and trichiasis, with corneal exposure of slight degree. Wearing corneal hard lens.

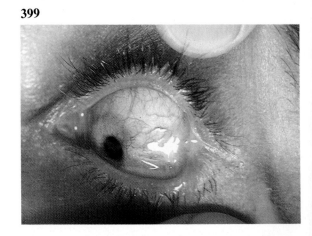

399

399 & 400 Metal burn and temporal symblepharon. After division the eye was treated with a scleral shell worn daily for three weeks. The rings are preferable and should be kept ready for use in several sizes and shapes.

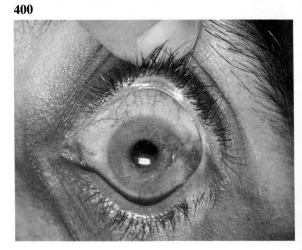

400

401–405 Treatment of symblepharon (Stevens–Johnson syndrome) by surgical division. Span of two years. To show use of ring and perfusion for several weeks and final fitting of a cosmetic shell. In Fig. 404 the cornea has cleaned sufficiently to diagnose 2° cataract.

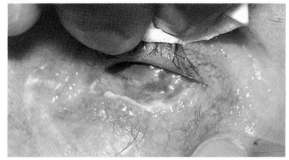

401

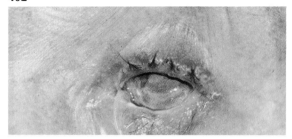

402

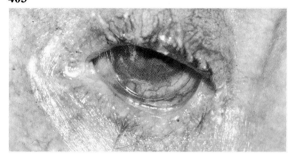

403

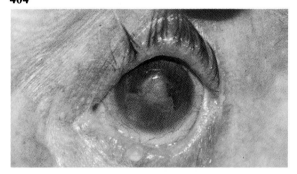

404

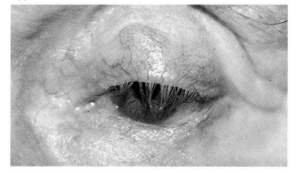

405

4. Adverse reactions to contact lens wear

Corneal reactions

406

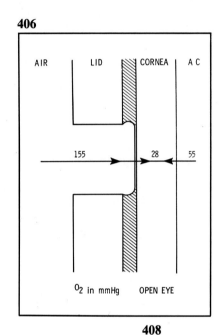

407

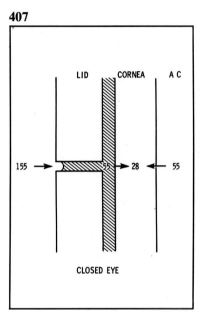

Gaseous exchange

406 With the lids open gases can be exchanged between the tear layer in front of the cornea and the atmosphere. The gradients of O_2 tensions are shown. CO_2 would show a gradient in the opposite direction (after I. Fatt).

407 With the lids closed gaseous exchange can occur via the capillaries of the lid palpebral conjunctivae. The contact lens will cause a relative degree of occlusion to both the above states.

408 The corneal surface uses 5μ 1cm^{-2} hour^{-1}. This is obtained from tears and atmosphere and from surrounding tissues, i.e. peripheral vessels, and aqueous. Nutritional molecules will also be supplied from similar sources.

409 The passage of O_2 through most materials is not directly related to the thickness of the lens. The graph shows that for PHEMA lenses thinner than 0.10mm the gas streams through at an increasing rate as the molecular thickness of the material is approached.

408

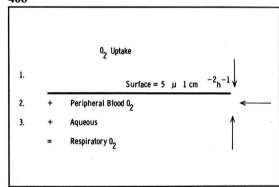

409

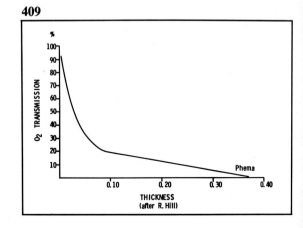

410 Gas transmission of materials. Different O_2 values of contact lens materials when compared with agar and water. Furthermore the rate increases by almost 20% if the temperature is changed from room (21°C) to the eye surface (33°C). The gas permeability of a lens made from a material is often different to the material transmissibility.

	O_2 transmission of materials (DK Units)	
	at 21°C	at 33°C
PHEMA	9.0	11.0
Sauflon 85 (CLM)	50	62
Duragel 75 (Cooper Lab)	40	49.6
'PERMA'	36	44.6
Agar	68	84.3
Water	78	96.7
Silicone rubber	100 to 600	100 to 600

411 O_2 uptake and the cornea. Uptake of O_2 from the surface of the cornea in comparison with that from a soft lens on the cornea. The slower fall off for a lens is due to the O_2 held by the lens.

412 & 413 Endothelial polymorphism. A contact lens wearer showed endothelial 'microcystic' lines in the endothelium. (Photography, R. Buckley.)

Specular applanation microscopy showed cellular polymorphism, possibly congenital. Not to be confused with 'Blebs' described by Holden and Zantos, which are caused by occlusion of rapid onset but resolving within an hour.

411

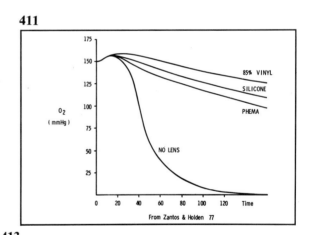

412

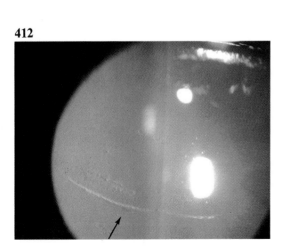

413

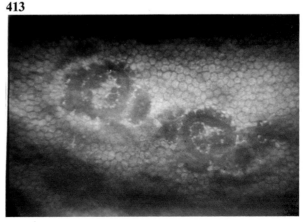

414 Epithelial mosaic. The contact lens rubs the tear lipid film off the epithelium and immediate removal of the lens can often show after fluorescein is installed a mosaic pattern of groups of superficial cells. (Photograph, A. Bron.)

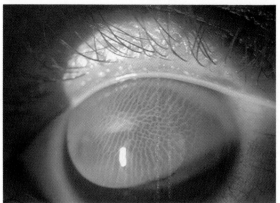

415 Epithelial oedema. To the left of the slit-beam is a dimpled pattern of the epithelium as seen by retro-illumination from iris reflection (soft lens wear).

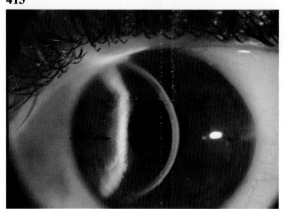

416 Tear film integrity. The lipid film is spread in waves (like wood grain) but the aqueous mucoid film is even surfaced. (Photograph, J-P. Guillon.) The aqueous-mucoid film can break where epithelial villi are damaged (black spots) or where drying rapidly occurs (break up zones). The latter provide a measurement of tear film quality. (Compare Figs. 499–501 of *Tear Film on Lens Surface* – Hamano *et al.*)

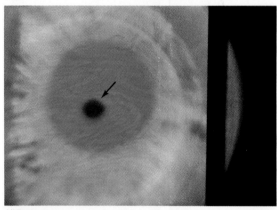

417 Tear film integrity. Surface bubbles and the normal lipid waves, suggesting areas of minimal lipid film over the mucous aqueous layer, the deeper part of which is held by the villi. (Photograph, J-P. Guillon.)

418 Tear film integrity. Lipid origin is from the meibomian gland orifice. (Photograph, J-P. Guillon.)

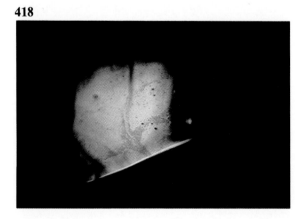

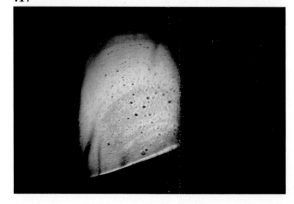

419a

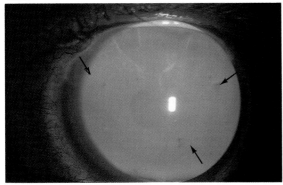

419b

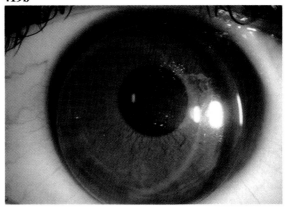

420

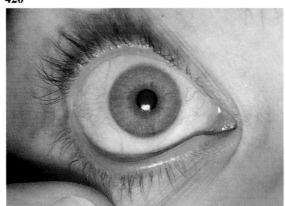

421

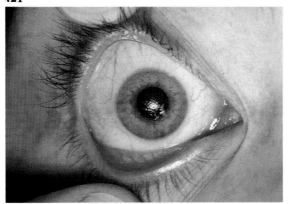

419a Tear film integrity. The tear film breaking up after four seconds always in the same area with identical pattern. (Photograph, Michel Guillon.)

Aetiology: either poor villi adhesion of deep mucoid-aqueous layer and/or rapid evaporation and poor lipid film cohesion.

419b The importance of normal tears with contact lens wearers cannot be overstressed. The photograph shows air bubbles trapped and remaining behind the lens because the tear surface tension is low.

420 & 421 Tear film and oedema. Tear film continuous over epithelial oedema after contact lens is removed showing early dimple pattern of superficial epithelial oedema (hard lens wear).

422 Corneal oedema. Similar oedema seen after wearing scleral lens for thyrotoxic eye.

N.B. Bubbles locate in the dimples.

423 Corneal oedema. High minus corneal contact lens which rides high and moves with upper lid showing localised oedema and dimple effect under sealed area.

423

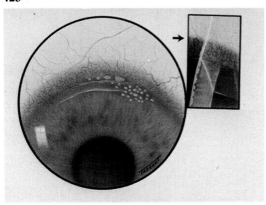

422

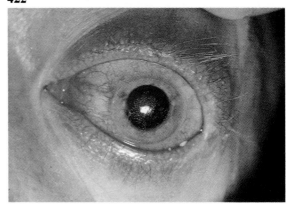

Superficial punctate keratitis. SPK.

424 Palpebral zone drying on either side of contact lens. Note conjunctival and superficial corneal epithelium punctate necrosis. Caused by dry eye problems, poor blinking or wearing in a dry environment.

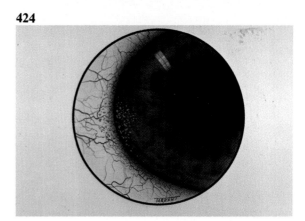

425 Central corneal superficial punctate keratitis from hard corneal contact lens wear.

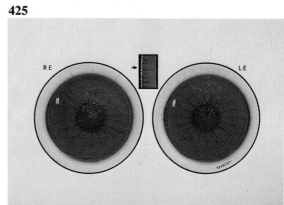

426 Haloes. Commonly seen with all types of contact lens wear. They are an interferometry phenomena. Oedema of cell layers or films on lenses will result in haloes.

Analysis: (1) from lens; (2) from corneal epithelium; (3) from crystalline lens; (4) from endothelium.

427 Granular superficial fibrillar keratitis. Hard lens wear caused the superficial changes combined with small epithelial cysts. These are either inter- or intra-cellular, most likely the latter. A common finding in all long-term contact lens wearers. A chronic change and often present for many months after cessation of wear. Does not decrease acuity in average patient.

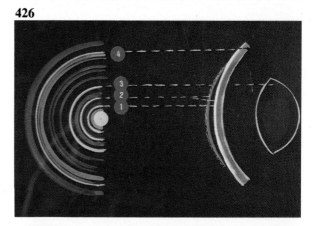

428 Aphakic cornea showing oedema. The patient wore hard corneal lenses, and SPK.

N.B. After operation corneal endothelium can easily decompensate.

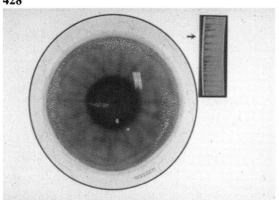

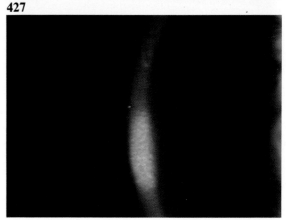

429 Dellen of stroma. Due to drying of cornea and seen with thick hard lens wear – not related to gas permeability of lens material.

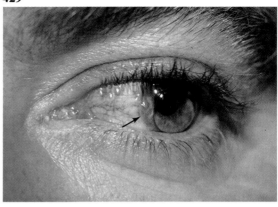

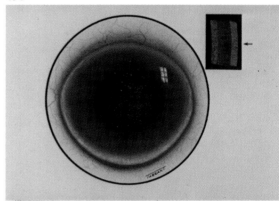

430 Aphakic cornea and punctate keratitis. Superficial epithelial oedema and punctate keratitis in an aphakic eye due to excessive thickness of lens. Note mostly central zone affected and traumatic in aetiology.

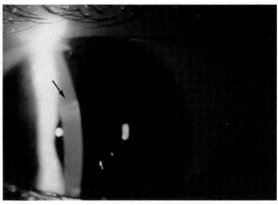

431 & 432 Superficial fibrillar changes. Very fine fibrillar changes in Bowman's layer in continuous wear soft hydrophilic lens (courtesy of Dr Stephani).

433 Corneal infiltrates. Several small infiltrates with vessels from continuous (extended) wear of gel lens.

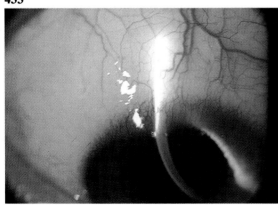

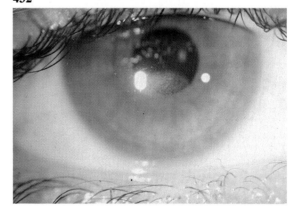

434 Corneal infiltration. Infiltrates (possible fibrillar and white cell deposits) in the Bowman's layers of the cornea with continuous wear gel lenses.

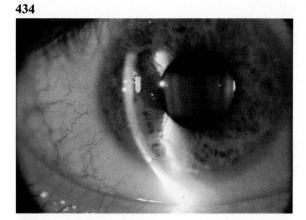

435 Stromal lysis. Inferior marginal stromal collagen lysis with continuous wear gel lens in aphakia.

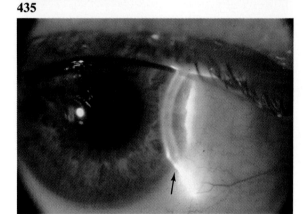

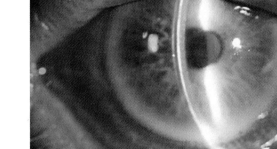

436 Occlusive lens syndrome. Occlusive gel lens syndrome after 24 hours wear, showing oedema of all corneal layers and endothelial Descemet folds and red eye. Same syndrome can occur after several successful months of gel lens wear.

Aetiology: hypo-secretion of tears or tight lens. Intra-ocular tension is often raised.

437 & 438 Central superficial keratitis. This is combined with papillary palpebral conjunctivitis from daily wear gel lenses of both eyes in this particular patient. Possible cold chemical disinfection sensitivity.

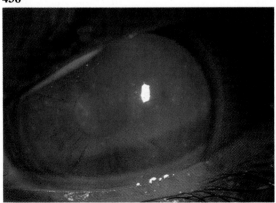

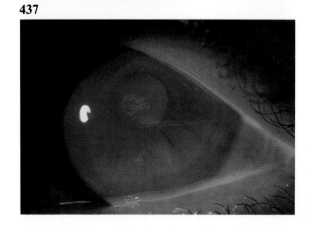

Neovascularisation of cornea

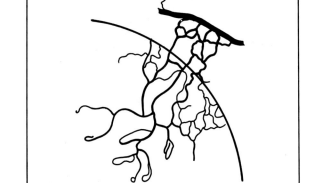

439 Diagrammatic outline of new corneal vessels from enlarged perilimbal end loops of capillaries.

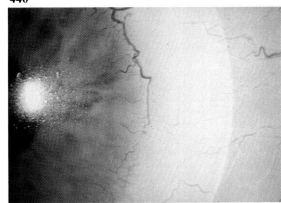

440 Neovascularisation of cornea in daily wear large gel lens.

N.B. Conjunctival vessels are *not* occluded by the lens.

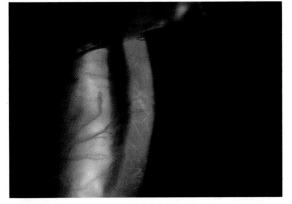

441 New vessels after several weeks of gel lens wear in dry eye problem.

442 Petechial corneal haemorrhages after occlusive soft lens wear.

443 Corneal vessels at all depths following two years of gel lens extended wear. Note fibrous plaques in stroma.

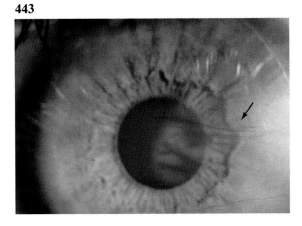

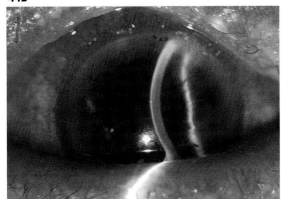

444

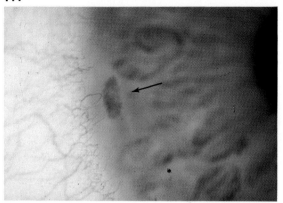

445

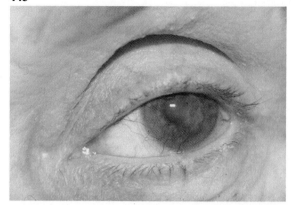

446

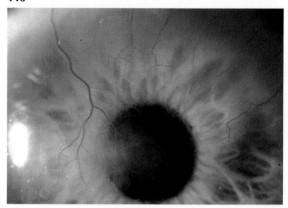

444 New corneal vessels in gel lens wear. *(Stromal.)*

445 Aphakic eye with new vessels and keratitis after extended wear of three months.

446 Keratoconus wearing scleral lenses (hard) 12 hours daily for several years with stromal vascularisation.

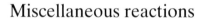

Miscellaneous reactions

447 Failed contact lens wear of all types due to dry eye problems. Note abnormal mucous adhesion to cornea – not Sjörgen's syndrome.

448 Dry eye wearer – reaction after a few hours of wear (gel lens). Possible chemical sensitivity.

449 Red eye, pain, blurred vision, sudden occlusive lens phenomena.

447

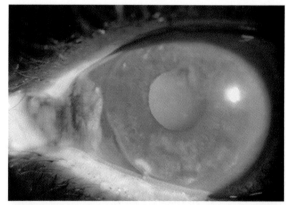

449

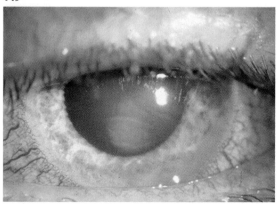

448

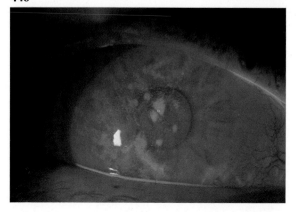

450 Sudden episode of occlusive lens phenomena in gel wearer after two years of successful wear. Note gross corneal oedema and folds in Descemets' membrane.

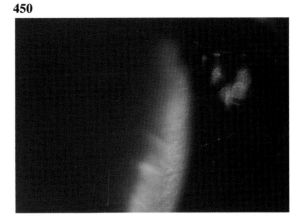

451 Pannus – in gel lens wearer (daily wear).

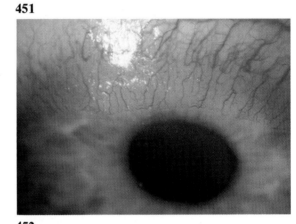

452 Uveitis. Uveitic response in young gel lens wearer (daily wear).

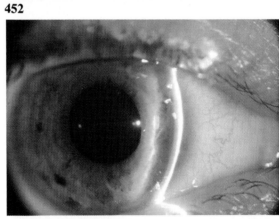

453 Endothelium. Early endothelial morphological changes in soft lens constant wear in young person after three years. *Low magnification.* (Photograph, N. Ahmed.)

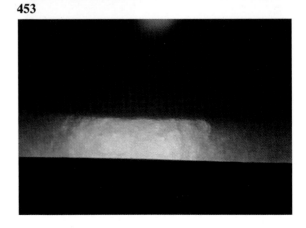

Optical problems

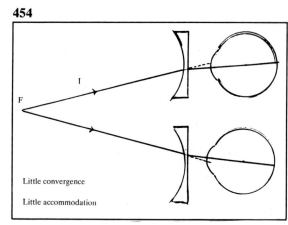

Little convergence

Little accommodation

454 Spectacles and myopia. Prismatic base in complementary near effect of spectacle minus lenses (myopia) may be a cause of convergence deficiency in contact lens wearer.

455 Accommodation. Myope wearing contact lenses has to accommodate more than spectacle wearer. (Drying of lens surface possibly biggest single cause of poor reading vision.)

455

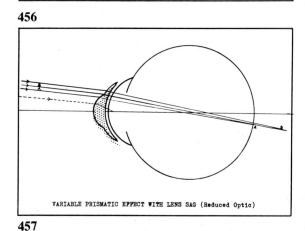

456 Reduced optics. High power and reduced optics in contact lenses can be cause of poor acuity, especially when poorly centred.

456

VARIABLE PRISMATIC EFFECT WITH LENS SAG (Reduced Optic)

457 'White Haloes'. Peripheral 'ghost' image formation due to contact lens edge or peripheral power distortion.

457

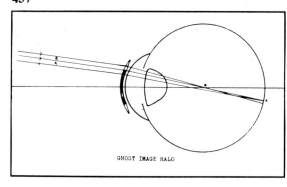

GHOST IMAGE HALO

Infective keratitis

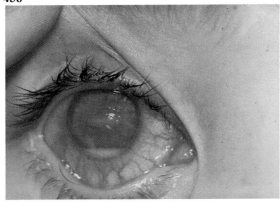

458

458 Riley-Day syndrome (familial dysautonomia) fitted with gel extended wear and resulting in hypopyon and pyocyaneus infection.

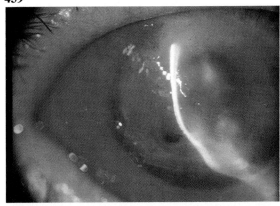

459

459 & 460 Pyocyaneus infection and hypopyon following extended wear lens and imperfect disinfection techniques.

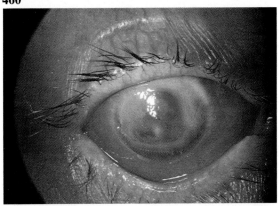

460

461 Extended wear aphakic eye and keratitis (*Staphylococcus* **infection).**

462 Fluorescein staining of previous eye.
N.B. Blue light shows up superficial lesions best.

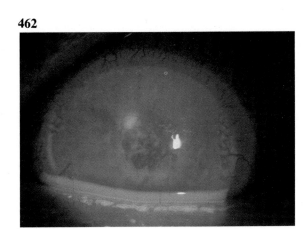

462

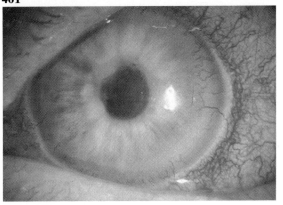

461

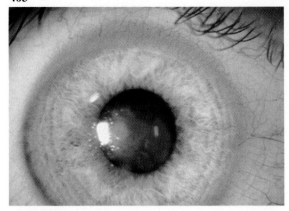

463 Infective keratitis and gel lens wear.

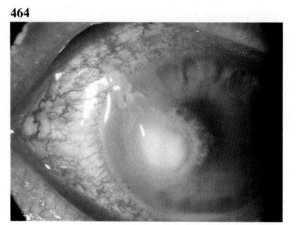

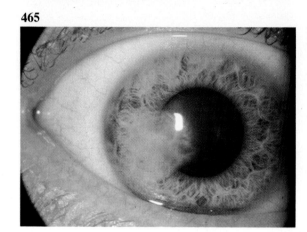

464 & 465 Pyocyaneus infection and extended gel wear. Same patient after six months.

466 The photokeratogram shows the degree of permanent corneal scarring. (Right eye.)

Right   Left

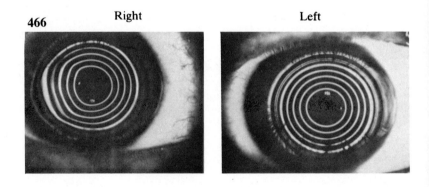

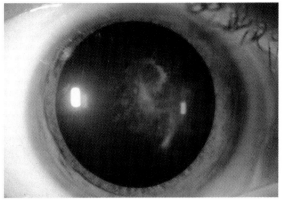

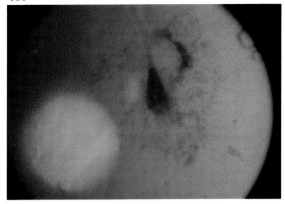

467 & 468 Infective keratitis in extended wear. Bacillus found in swab of conjunctiva. Retro-illumination of affected cornea.

469 Daily wear gel lens. Onset of problem after three years of wear. Bacillus grown from eye. △ nummular keratitis.

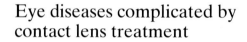

Eye diseases complicated by contact lens treatment

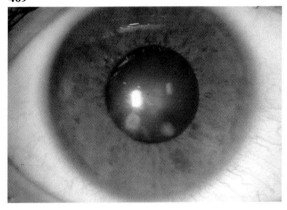

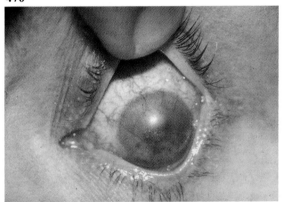

470 & 471 Trachoma (quiescent). Complicated by wearing high water content soft lens (65%) showing extensive new vessels and drying of lens. Same eye one year later (Fig. 471) and six months after graft operation. Now wearing silicone rubber contact lens 10.80mm diameter. successfully.

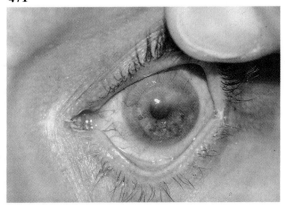

472a

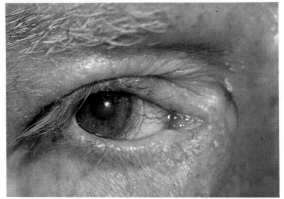

472b

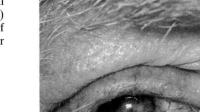

472a & b, 473 **Exposure keratitis** from VIIth cranial nerve palsy with soft lens fitting (had worn scleral hard) at commencement of wear. Same eye. Nine months of continuous wear gel lens. Vessel and infiltration of scar tissue after two years of gel lens wear.

473

474

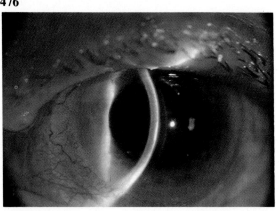

474 & 475 **Exposure keratitis.** Before contact lens fitting of exposure keratitis due to VIIth cranial nerve palsy. High water content gel lens wear some six months later showing vascularisation and fibrosis of cornea.

N.B. Patient now wearing scleral hard lens.

476 **Aphakia.** Aphakic eye fitted with 85% water content gel lens at end of operation. Central corneal epithelial necrosis occurred on seventh day after operation.

476

475

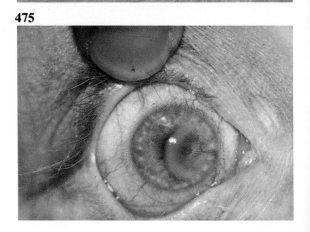

477 Aphakia and endothelium. Endothelial density deficiency morphological abnormalities in aphakic eye. Cell density and/or corneal thickness should be known before extended wear commences and be reassessed if problems occur.

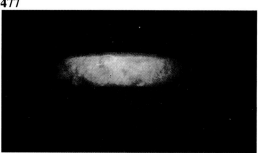

478 & 479 Aphakic bullous keratopathy. Eye fitted successfully with gel bandage lens for over one year. Onset of red eye with infection four days after lens was cleaned, sterilised and replaced. Is aetiology due to disruption of mucous film on lens from the cleaning process?

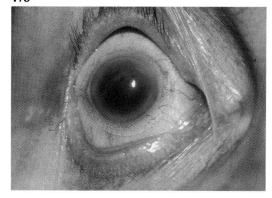

480a Desensitization of superficial cornea. A trephine is used to cut down to half stromal thickness.

480b Adhesive contact lens and epikeratoplasty. Adhesives and lens materials are to toxic for permanent contact lens fixation but H. Kaufman has used the method to correct aphakia with human donor cornea and sutures.

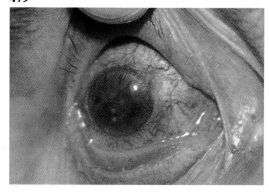

481 Keratoconus corneal desensitization. To trephine cuts to half corneal thickness of 5mm and 10mm diameter followed by successful hard lens wear.

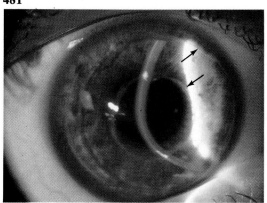

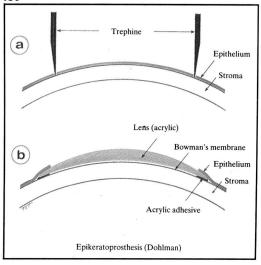

482 Keratoconus and intolerance to contact lens. Radial keratectomy in keratoconic cornea producing a small degree of corneal flattening and improving contact lens tolerance.

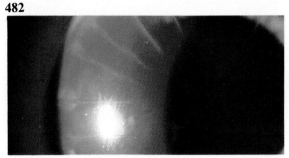

483 Hydrops keratoconus. Hydrops in keratoconus, e.g. wearing hard contact lens. Aetiology from Descemet's rupture following eye rubbing or removing contact lens with excessive pressure.

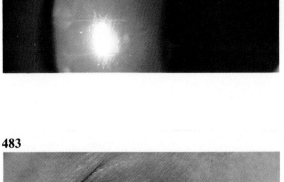

484 Hydrops keratoconus. Hydrops in keratoconus wearing contact lens as seen from the side.

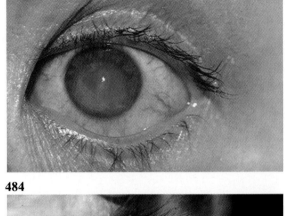

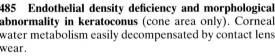

485 Endothelial density deficiency and morphological abnormality in keratoconus (cone area only). Corneal water metabolism easily decompensated by contact lens wear.

N.B. also seen in keratoplasty.

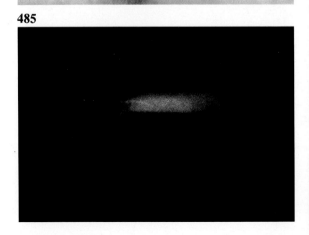

Lids and conjunctival complications

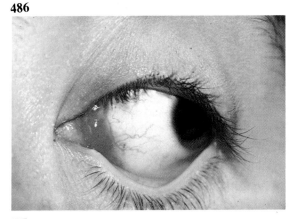

486 Caruncle. Infection of caruncle associated with contact lens wear.

487 Sclera. Trauma from scleral lens causing conjunctivitis.

488 Blepharitis and lid oedema from contact lens wear problem.

488

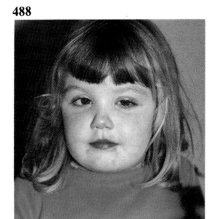

487

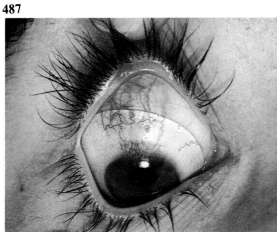

489

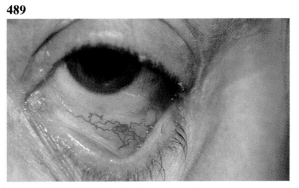

489 Blepharitis with sebaceous deposits on lashes. Note chronic palpebral hyperaemia.

490

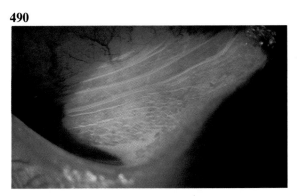

490 Conjunctivitis. Papillary pattern slightly exaggerated to show conjunctival wrinkles.

491

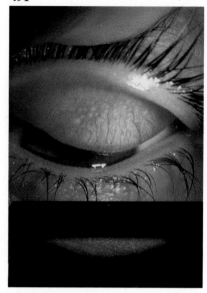

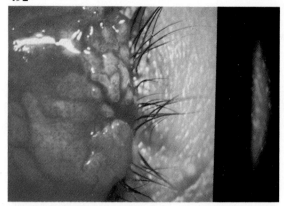
492

493

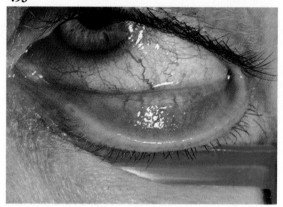

491 Conjunctivitis. Hard follicle formation – lymphoid response to chronic contact lens irritation.

492 Vernal conjunctivitis. Gross papillary reaction to soft lens wear – latent vernal conjunctivitis. (Photograph, R. Pearce.)

493 Conjunctivitis. Acute conjunctival lymphoid response to contact lens solutions.

494

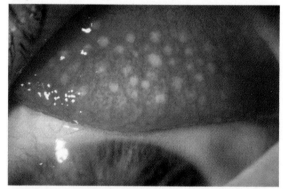

494 Chronic follicular and papillary conjunctivitis. A chronic response to several years' wear of PMMA lens.

495

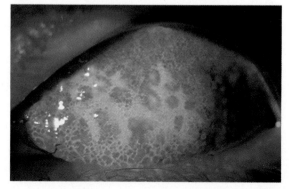

495 Chronic follicular and papillary conjunctivitis. The fluorescein drop shows the papillary outline confined to the fornicular conjunctivae. A papillary response in the tarsal plate is more common with vernal catarrhal conjunctivitis.

496 & 497 Histology of contact lens conjunctivitis.
Papillae in histological section from biopsy of patient
with moderate lymphoid and hypertropic reaction. Note
excessive mucoid cells and inflammatory cell invasion
and vessels in deeper tissues. Mast cells evident at higher
magnification are typical of allergic immunological
aetiology of papillary conjunctivitis.

496

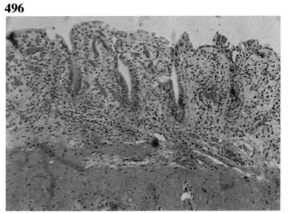

497

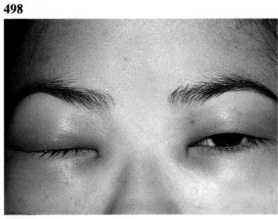

498

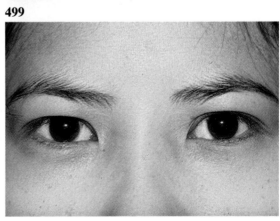

498 Allergy reaction. Allergic lid reaction to new solution.

499 Allergy reaction. Five days later after withdrawal
of contact lens wear.
    Reaction recurred with old lenses and solutions – new
lenses and heat/saline produced *no* reaction.

5. Contact lens spoilation

The aetiology is of several sources.

Surface texture:
  Loss of integrity of finish
  Loss of curvature
  Change in size and shape and thickness
  Tears.

Surface deposits:
  Tear secretions – lipids, mucous, etc.
  Tissue debris – cells
  Enzyme activity
  Salts
  Micro-organisms.

Lens substance:
  Polymer blemishes and degeneratives
  Polymer linkage breakdown – physical changes
  Colour change
  Water absorption and transparency changes.

500

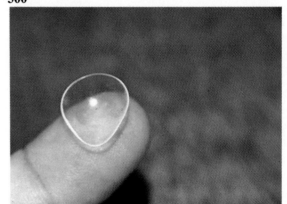

500 Irregular shape. The lens material after use may undergo changes in elasticity and plasticity irregularly, resulting in warped form.

501

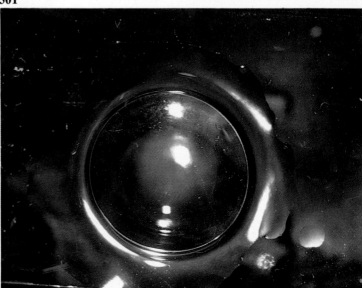

501 Amorphous white discolouration. The white deposits are not due to micro-organisms, but to loss of transparency caused by polymer changes.

502 Brown discolouration. A very common change of colour and sometimes associated with increased rigidity. The gel lens may absorb tyrosine from tears or even dyes from the human tears. Some lenses become brown if the material is incompletely polymerised or contains additives.

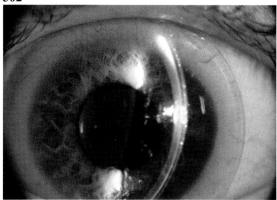

503 Ultraviolet spectrometry. The peaks suggest that one or two substances of protein type may be causing discolouration. Minerals such as magnesium, chromium, manganese in very small concentration will cause permanent lens discolouration. (A. Winder.)

503

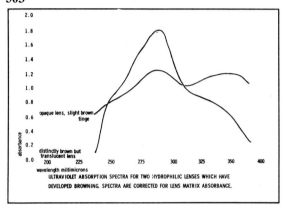

ULTRAVIOLET ABSORPTION SPECTRA FOR TWO HYDROPHILIC LENSES WHICH HAVE DEVELOPED BROWNING. SPECTRA ARE CORRECTED FOR LENS MATRIX ABSORBANCE.

504 Surface granular deposits. These surface deposits contain little if any lipid or mucin as compared with Figs. 529 and 530. They are associated with dry eye problems.

504

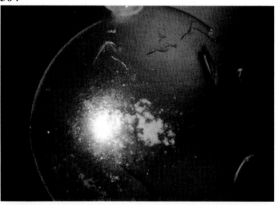

505 Plastic degeneration – white. Polymer degradation will result sometimes in water absorption and loss of transparency due to irregular break up of the molecular chains. The area swells and appears white or grey.

506 Silicone rubber lens deposits. The siloxane material adheres selectively to lipids and where the lens surface loses its hydrophilic properties, drying also rapidly occurs. The illustration shows rapidly drying area which can have abrasive problems.

N.B. Siloxane can transmit water vapour.

506

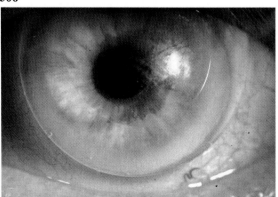

505

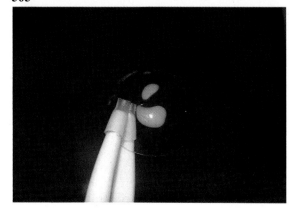

507 Lipid deposits on silicone rubber lenses. The conglomerate of lipid and muco-protein is smooth and regularly curved and is not the same as the 'mulberry' complex (Fig. 529 & 530) seen on hydrophilic lens surfaces. The later deposits form about a nidus of polymer degeneration. The silicone rubber deposit adheres to non-hydrophilic dry areas of the lens surface.

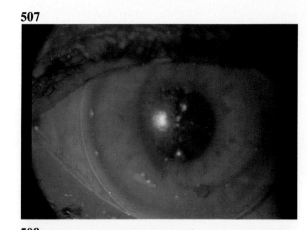

508 & 509 Dry areas on silicone rubber lenses. The aphakic eye wears these lenses continuously often for several weeks. The dry eye deposits accumulate until vision is seriously obscured. They appear to be altered lipid plus protein secretions dried on the lens surface.

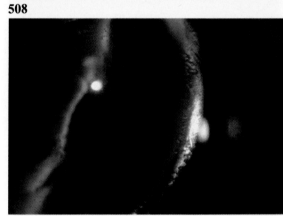

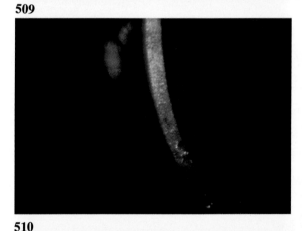

510–512 White discrete deposits. These deposits were shown to be calcium salts in a normal young female PHEMA (38%) wearer. They occurred after only one or two weeks of wear and were controlled only by soaking the lenses at night in EDTA 1% solution. The tears were shown to have an abnormal Ca level.

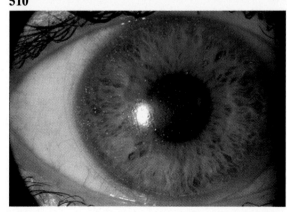

511

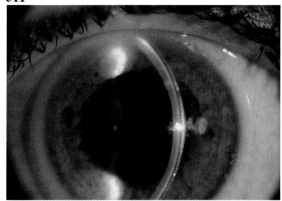

512

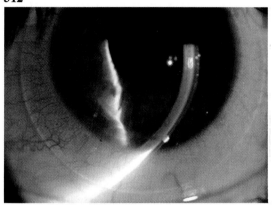

513

513 Analysis of deposits can be done by micro-atomic probe, atomic spectrometer, selective dyes and histo-chemical techniques with ultra microscopy of the lenses. The read-out concerns micro-probe atomic analysis of lens subtrates showing calcium and phosphate present and their relative concentrations.

514 Analysis of deposits. This slide of the lens substance shows by selective staining that calcium salt crystals are mostly at the surface but also in the lens substance (R. Tripathi).

515 & 516 Grey and white gelatinous degeneration. Two examples of lenses worn continuously and areas of gelatinous plastic degeneration occurred.

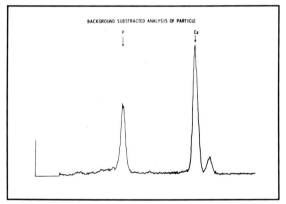

515

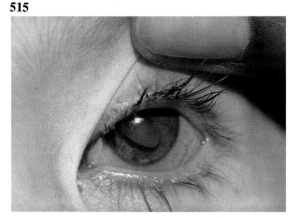

514

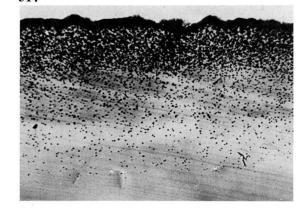

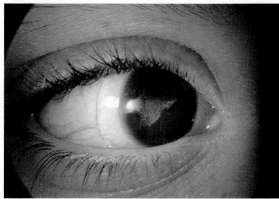

517 Phase contrast microscopy. Using low power magnification and polarised light the lens surface can be examined in saline and other solutions without damaging the lens. This photograph shows the quality of a CAB lens. This material absorbed 3% water by weight. Note the granular appearance of the surface and the similarity with other contact lens surfaces.

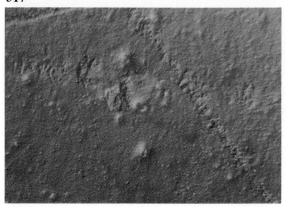

518 Phase contrast of hydrophilic gel lens surface. Granular surface fractures and also depressions. The surfaces of some elevations have broken down and are filled with deposits.

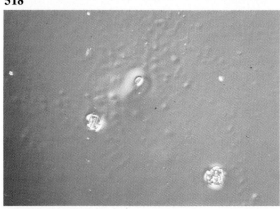

519 Phase contrast of gel lens surface deposits (iron). The deposit is most likely iron and some other metal chemically attached to lipid and adherent to the polymer. This lipo-chemical deposit is in a cone of poor surface polymerisation as denoted by the irregular circular depression.

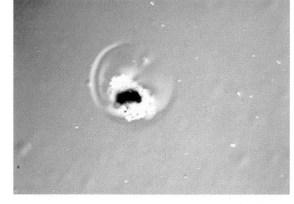

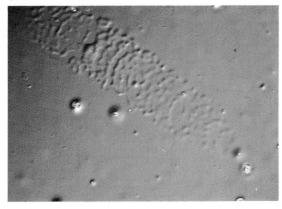

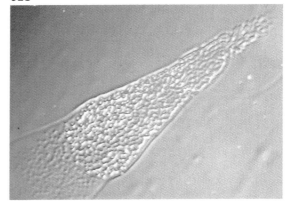

520 Polymerisation defect (moulded lens – gel). The surface shows a large zone of uneven polymerisation causing irregular ridges and waves on the surface. (Moulded Lens.)

521 Polymerisation defect. Another example of surface polymer defect. (Moulded Lens.)

522 Striae at edge – phase contrast. The material is possibly under stress at the periphery and shows loss of homogenicity.

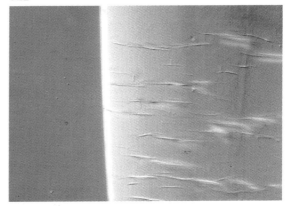

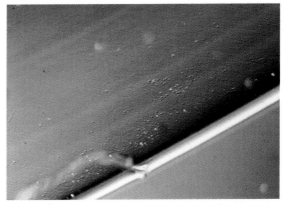

523 Breakage at edge. A tear in the edge not seen with the naked eye.

524 Wetting of the surface. The ability of a lens surface to wet with tears and form a continuous film is the most important single factor for optical function and tolerance of a lens. Hydrophilic properties of the substance do not necessarily relate to wetting properties of the surface. The photograph shows how saline spreads on a silicone rubber lens surface. The droplets are small and separate. *(× 50)*

525 Wetting of the surface. The hydrated 75% lens (amino-amide) shows larger areas of confluent saline than in the previous photograph of silicone rubber lens.

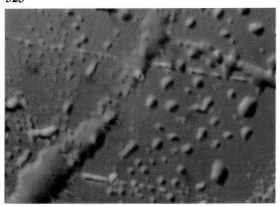

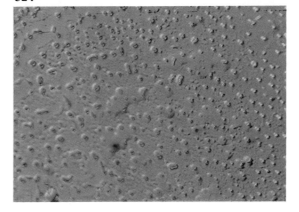

526

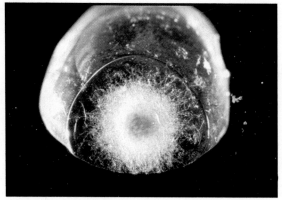

527

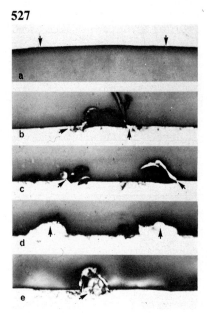

526 Yeast and fungus infections of lenses. A neglected unused hydrophilic lens found to have a total growth of fungus after four days.

527 & 528 Microscopy of extended wear gel lens (65% water). (a) Arrows indicate intact front surface of lens; (b), (c), (d), (e) the back surface is broken up in several areas as shown by the arrows. The patient developed keratitis after two months of wear. (Section by R. Tripathi.)

A very high magnification shows an area of surface degeneration with micro-organism, most likely yeast type (arrow).

528

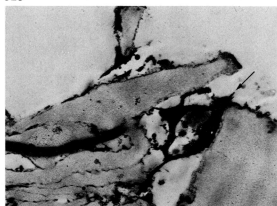

529 & 530 Mucoid deposits on hydrophilic gel lenses (daily wear). These gel deposits follow a conglomerate pattern (mulberry).

530

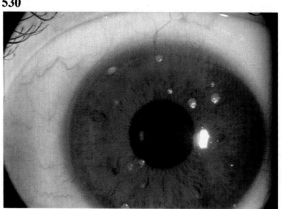

529

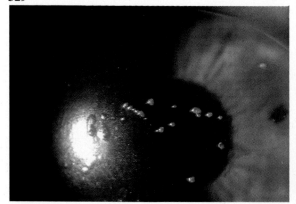

531a & b–534 **Muco-lipid deposits.** The high magnifications show the lipid as bifringent optical density and in Fig. 533 the lipid is seen to form laminar concentric patterns scattered with calcium deposits and supported by micro-protein. Fig. 534 shows an early polymer nidus of a conglomerate. (All these preparations were made by R. & B. Tripathi.)

531a

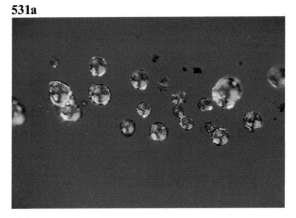

531b

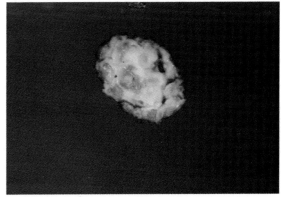

532

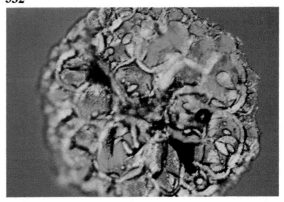

534

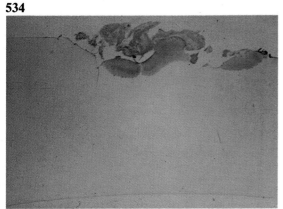

533

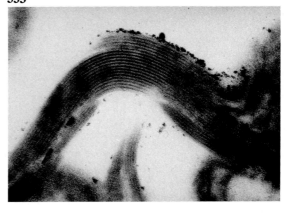

535 Lens surface tear films. Using a differential inter-ference technique as used for static lens surface examination, i.e. phase contrast, Hamano, Kawabe, Umeno, Mitsunaga and Onishi, showed the details of lipid and micro-protein films on the cornea and lens surface *in situ*. The same detail can be seen using white oblique illumination (J-P. Guillon) and very simple instrumentation. The conventional use of the slit-beam microscope has prevented users from making these observations hitherto. The tear film as seen on the new PMMA lens. The lipid waves are regular and eddy around debris. To the left a front is formed about a dry area. (cf Fig. 525.)

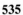
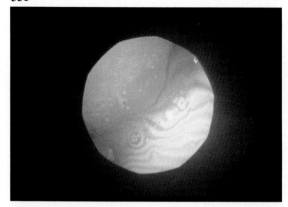

536 Lens surface tear films (Hamano *et al*). The tear film will not flow on to the rough surface covered by debris. No lipid waves are noted (marble graining).

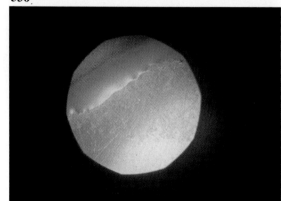

537 Lens surface tear films (Hamano *et al*). The tear film as seen on a hydrophilic gas permeable hard lens surface is relatively normal. The lipid waves are regular and *no* eddying around isolated zones is seen.

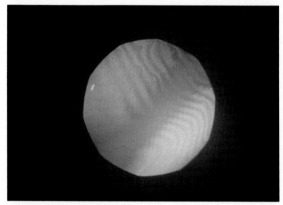

538 Lens and lens surface contamination. A lens (gel) surface contaminated by micro-organisms. *Pseudomonas* was found in the lens case.

539 Lens and lens surface contamination. A lens showing mycelium in the surface.

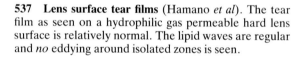

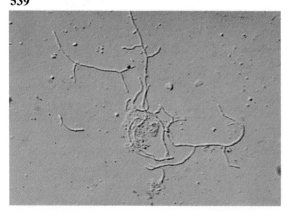
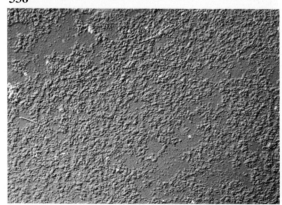

540

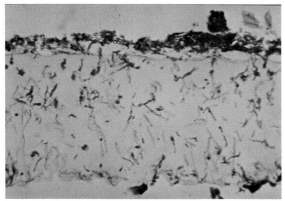

542

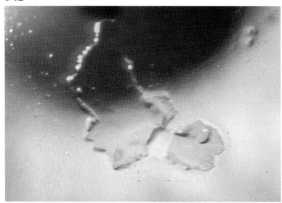

543

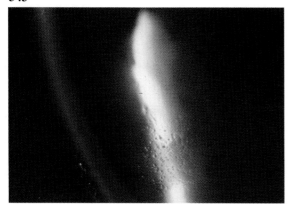

544

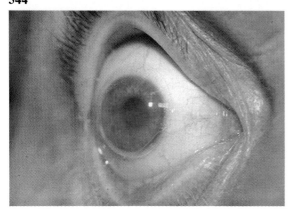

541

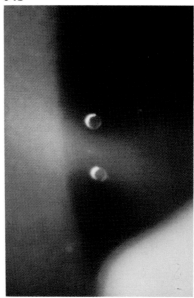

540 Lens and lens surface contamination. A lens showing mycelium in its substance.

541 Lens cystic degeneration. Breakdown of polymer occurred after three weeks' use of the lens.

542 Surface imperfection. After wearing a gel (38%) for six months, an area of the surface peeled away.

543 Drying of lens *in situ*. A toric gel with prism base down truncation was not covered by the lids whilst worn. The surface drying results in deposits and a granular appearance.

544 Drying of lens *in situ*. The inferior zone of a spherical gel lens elevates from the eye surface when dry – the lens can eventually fall off the eye if drying proceeds.

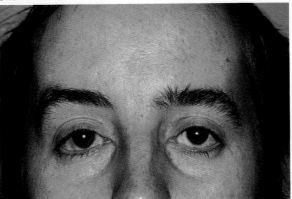

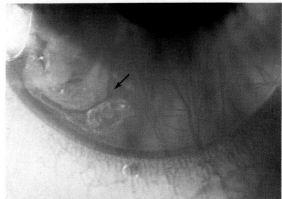

545 & 546   Myotonic dystrophy and stagnation of tear flow with scleral lens wear. This case illustrates that in the absence of regular blinking the tear flow behind a scleral lens is not possible. The muco-protein precipitates as gelatinous stringy deposits. This patient also shows hypoxia and corneal neovascularisation.

N.B. Fitted to elevate the lid.

6. Prosthetics

547 Types of ocular prosthetics.

Top left – opaque white haptic, coloured optic and black pupil.

Top right – clear haptic, tinted optic.

Bottom left – opaque white haptic, tinted clear blue optic.

Bottom right – opaque optic iris, clear optic pupil, clear haptic.

Centre – clear haptic, iris and pupil opaque.

The above examples are made in PMMA material, vegetable and oil paint laminates. But soft plastics can be used in some examples and usually round shapes.

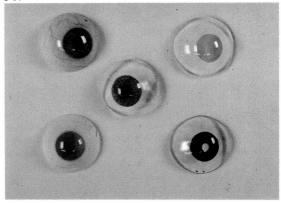

547

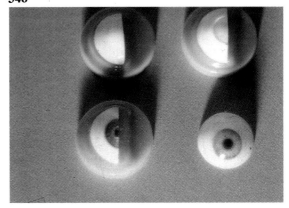

548

548 Stages in manufacture of a prosthetic shell or prosthesis.

Corneal lens prosthetics

549 Corneal lenses with iris tinting.

550 Corneal lens with iris pattern.

551 Occlusive lens of corneal size.

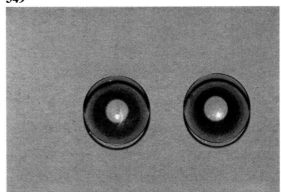

549

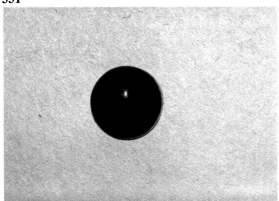

551

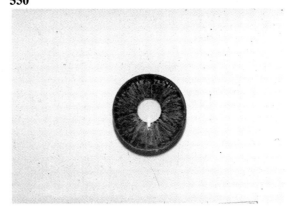

550

Shell
prosthetics

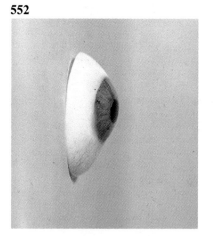

552 Shell prosthesis of hard material.

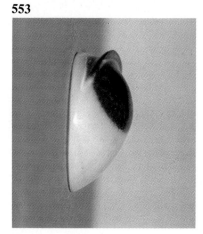

553 **Lid ledge.** Shell prosthesis for ptosis correction.

554–556 **Shell prosthesis for a divergent blind eye.**
With spectacles which can be used to magnify or minify the affected eye and even use a prism on one side only to produce best cosmetic effect.

554

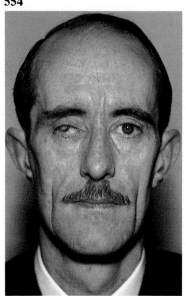

555

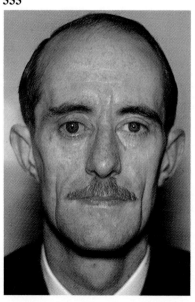

556

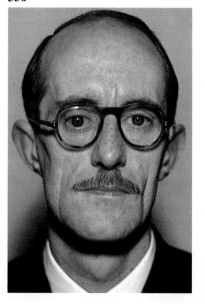

557 & 558 Prosthesis for a divergent blind eye. Dermoid. Shell prosthesis for a blind eye.

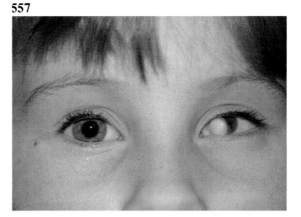

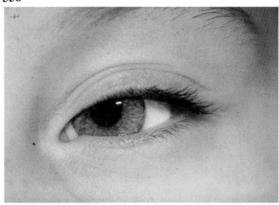

559 & 560 Convergent blind eye. Convergent blind right eye in child with coloured hard shell.

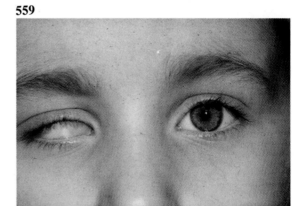

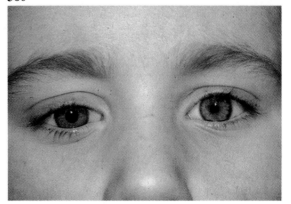

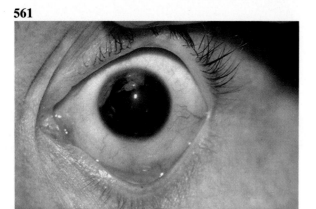

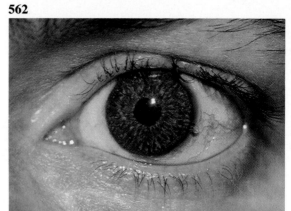

561 & 562 Secondary aniridia. Cosmetic lens for traumatic aniridia in a very photosensitive eye.

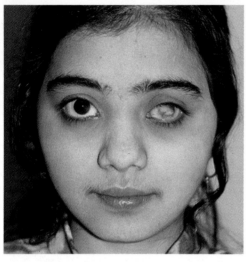

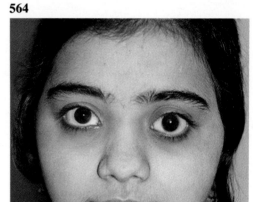

563 & 564 Child's eye prosthesis. Child with blind eye following infection fitted with cosmetic shell.

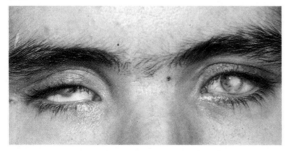

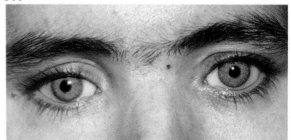

565 & 566 Bilateral corneal leucomata eyes from birth infection fitted with shells and clear pupils because patient has perception of light.

567 & 568 Albino. To occlude light and correct astigmatism.

N.B. High astigmatism is common in ocular albinism. Also note photophobia and wish to close eyes without contact lenses (Fig. 567).

567

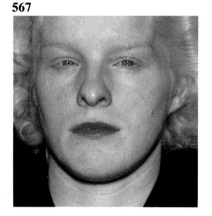

568

569

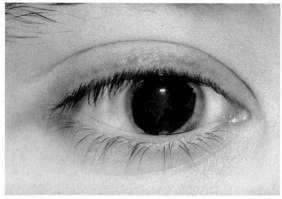

570

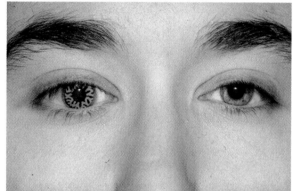

569 & 570 Traumatic aniridia. Right eye fitted with corneal hard lens (Nusyte) with coloured iris and optical correction.

571

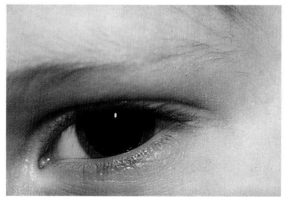

572

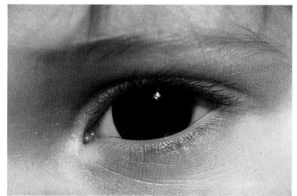

571 & 572 Congenital aniridia. Fitted with hydrophilic iris coloured lenses (Weicon).

573 & 574 Iris colomba from injury. Eye fitted with iris print (Weicon) in hydrophilic soft lens, copied from photograph slide.

N.B. Where a good match is not possible both eyes can be fitted with coloured soft lenses of the same colour.

Colour prints using photography can be applied to some soft materials.

573

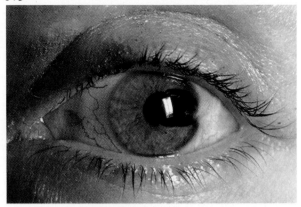

574

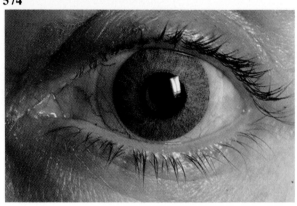

575 & 576 Blind eye fitted with tinted soft lenses. (Igel Optics)

575

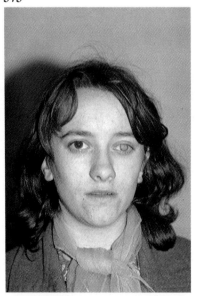

576

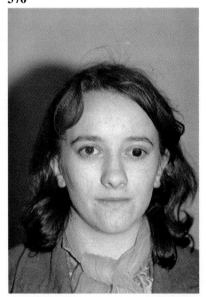

577 & 578 **Opaque pupil in a gel lens** to occlude vision in patient with insuperable diplopia.

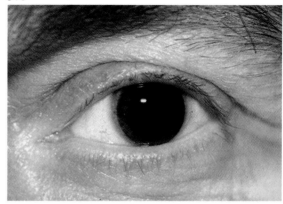

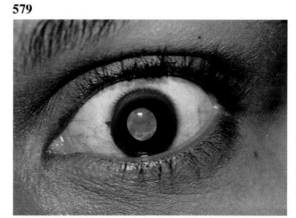

579 & 580 **Tinted gel lens** used to mask inoperable cataract. (Igel Optics)

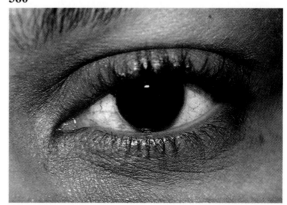

Orbital prosthesis – artificial eyes

The prosthesis can be fitted by:
 1. Making a model from an orbital impression (*see* scleral lens, page 23) and Figs. 581–583) or 2. modifying half spherical back surface shaped eyes (Figs. 542–595).

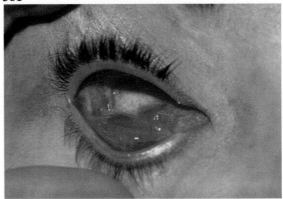

581   Socket with buried implant.

Moulded prosthesis

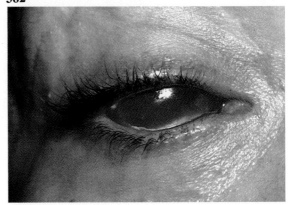

582   **Clear acrylic** fitted and to be marked for pupil centre and iris size, etc. (made from an impression of the socket).

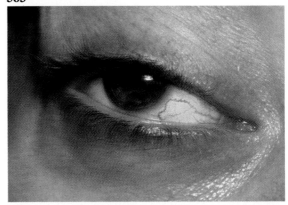

583   Finished artificial eye in socket.

A common problem

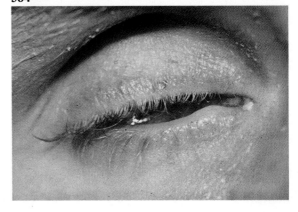

584 & 585   **Deep superior groove** due to orbital fat atrophy and retraction of levator. Note inferior ectropion.

140

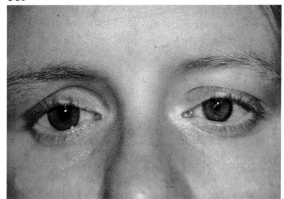

585 Best prosthesis possible.

Preformed artificial eyes

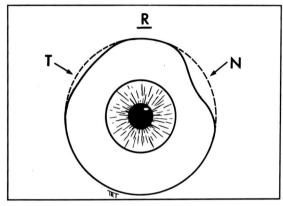

586 Diagram of an artificial eye shape. (Note the nasal indentation and △ shape.)

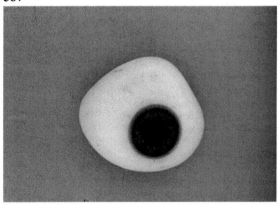

587 One eye from a set to show ⚠ shape with nasal notch. This shape prevents rotation.

588–591 The diagrams illustrate areas of a prosthesis which can be modified either to centre a prosthesis (1–4), or to fill in superior lid grooves (6).

These modifications are done by adding wax and then reproducing the prosthesis or by taking away substance.

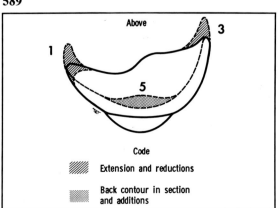

589

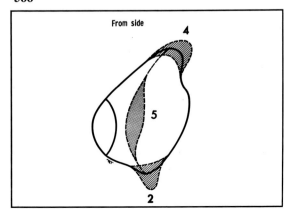

588

590

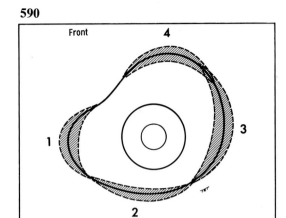

591

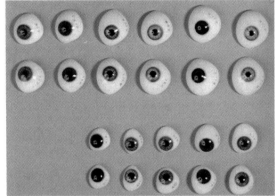

592

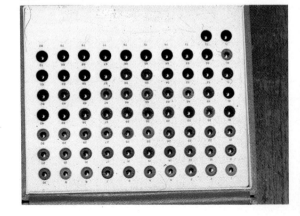

592 A set of artificial trial eyes – (Nissel Artificial eye).

593 Master scleral colours for matching – (Nissel Artificial eye).

594 Master iris colours for matching – (Nissel Artificial eye).

594

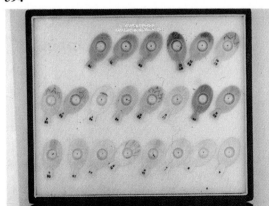

593

595 Scleral colour with iris match *in situ* – (Nissel Artificial eye).

595

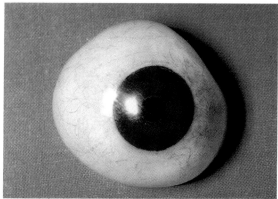

Fitting of the preformed shape

596 Artificial eye. A prosthesis (right).

596

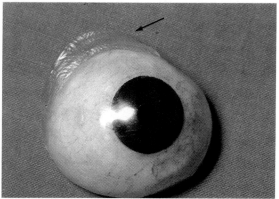

597 The prosthesis *in situ* (right) and formed to be divergent.
N.B. Left is also a prosthesis. Bilateral anophthalmia.

598 Right prosthesis modified with wax and then remade.

599 Further wax modification.

600 Final result.

597

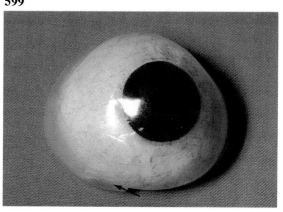

598

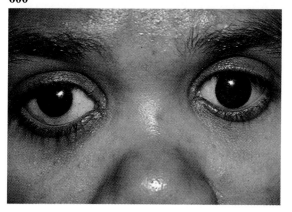

599

600

601–603 Artificial eyes. Plastic surgery to modify the socket (plastic inclusions) or to correct ectropion is advised in some cases. This photograph shows lower ectropia with temporal gaping. Hitching of the lower tarsal plate to the upper inner lid (resected) produces normal appearance. Diagram of ectropia correction (Fig. 603).

601

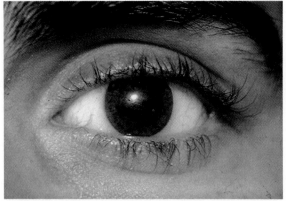

603

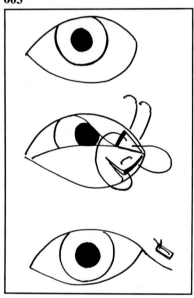

602

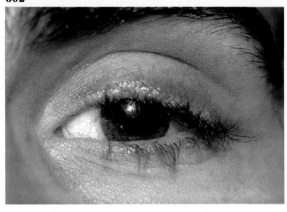

604 Artificial eyes – Anophthalmia. Bilateral congenital anophthalmia. Funicular sockets. Blepharophimosis.

605 Artificial eyes. Fitted with black beads as initial procedure. In babies a series of black beads of increasing size must be used until the socket is sufficiently large to take a coloured prosthesis soft materials can be used suitably dyed.

604

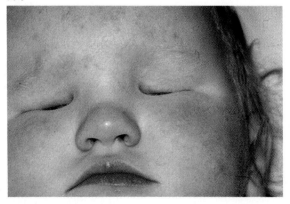

605

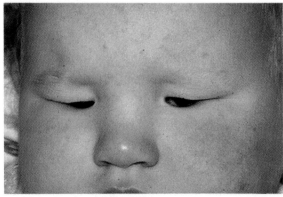

Index

Index

References are to picture and caption numbers.